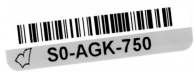

Self-Interest and Universal Health Care

Self-Interest
and Universal
Health Care

Why Well-Insured
Americans Should
Support Coverage
for Everyone

LARRY R. CHURCHILL

Harvard University Press
Cambridge, Massachusetts
London, England
1994

Copyright © 1994 by the President and Fellows of Harvard College
All rights reserved
Printed in the United States of America

This book is printed on acid-free paper, and its binding
materials have been chosen for strength and durability.

Library of Congress Cataloging-in-Publication Data
Churchill, Larry R., 1945–
Self-interest and universal health care : Why well-insured
Americans should support coverage for everyone / Larry R. Churchill.
p. cm.
Includes bibliographical references and index.
ISBN 0-674-80092-3
1. Right to health care—United States. 2. Insurance, Health—
Government policy—United States. 3. Health services
accessibility—United States. 4. Health care reform—United States.
I. Title.
RA395.A3C495 1994
362.1'0973—dc20
94-14568
CIP

For Shelley and Blair

Contents

Acknowledgments

I have many people and organizations to thank for their help and encouragement in bringing this volume to fruition.

In 1991 I was fortunate to receive three years of support from the Charles E. Culpeper Foundation by being designated a Scholar in the Medical Humanities. This funding released me from teaching and administration for brief but productive periods over the past three years, and made possible travel and research assistance. I am most grateful for this support.

During the summer of 1992 I was a Visiting Fellow of the Institute for Advanced Studies in the Humanities at the University of Edinburgh. Here I found receptive conversation partners for my work on David Hume and Adam Smith and a commodious environment in which to work. I want to thank especially Peter Jones, the director of the institute, for his interest in the project, and Vincent Hope of the Department of Philosophy for our conversations and for his critical appraisal of my interpretations of sympathy.

In the spring of 1992 I was invited to give the George Washington Gay Lecture at Harvard Medical School, and this provided an occasion to present some of my ideas about the role of self-interest in health care reform. I thank especially Lynn Peterson, who was my host for the Gay Lectureship, and Rashi Fein, who challenged me to better formulations of my thesis.

Various drafts of this manuscript have been typed by three dedicated and skilled persons. Angela Boudwin suffered through the preliminary drafts, Delores Musselman the penultimate ones; finally, I have been fortunate to have the able and energetic assistance of Becky Eatmon. All have my appreciation and thanks.

Allan Brandt helped me to sort out some of the ideas in Chapters 3 and 5, and provided his usual encouragement. Nancy King read some of the early drafts and sharpened my prose. Fifteen years of conversations with Glenn Wilson on health policy and social justice have shaped my thinking in pervasive ways; it would be hard to itemize them or overestimate their importance. Loretta Kopelman made some timely and adroit criticisms of my application of Hume to health policy. I am very grateful for the assistance of each of these friends and colleagues. More generally, I owe a great deal to the intellectual community of the University of North Carolina at Chapel Hill gathered together in the Department of Social Medicine. I feel fortunate to be a part of it.

Marion Danis co-authored an earlier version of the parts of Chapter 5 that concern citizenship; I am appreciative for that collaboration and additional ones since. Barry Saunders served as my research assistant during 1991–92. That year of conversations with him about Hume and Smith deepened my understanding and was of enormous help in clarifying the perspective taken in this volume. As always, the most consistently insightful help has come from my spouse, Sande. No acknowledgment here can tell the full story of this indebtedness, nor of my gratitude.

Finally, I want to thank two persons at Harvard University Press. Michael Fisher was a consistent source of help in guiding this volume to publication, while the editorial skills of Kate Schmit made every page better than it would have been otherwise.

I dedicate this book to my daughters, Shelley and Blair, in the hope that their generation will enjoy a more just social compact for health care.

This book contains reworked materials from the following essays: "Private Virtues, Public Detriment: Allocating Scarce Medical Resources to the Elderly," *Ethics*, 100:1 (1989), pp. 169–176, © 1989 by the University of Chicago, all rights reserved; "Theories of Justice," in *Ethical Problems in Dialysis and Transplantation*, edited by Carl M. Kjellstrand and John B. Dossetor (Dordrecht:

Kluwer Academic Publishers, 1992), pp. 26–31, © 1992 Kluwer Academic Publishers, reprinted by permission of Kluwer Academic Publishers; "Getting from 'I' to 'We'," in *A Good Old Age?* edited by Paul Homer and Martha Holstein (New York: Simon and Schuster, 1990), pp. 109–119; "Realigning Our Thinking in Health Care: What Are Our Rights and Responsibilities?" in *North Carolina Insight*, 13:3–4, pp. 109–113, published by the North Carolina Center for Public Policy Research, Raleigh, North Carolina; and "Autonomy and the Common Weal," co-authored with Marion Danis, *Hastings Center Report*, 21:1 (1991), pp. 25–31. I thank Marion Danis and the editors and publishers of these publications for granting permission to reprint sections of these essays here.

Self-Interest and Universal Health Care

Introduction

The conventional wisdom about the U.S. health care system is that it suffers from two chronic problems: escalating costs and limited access. Repeated analyses of health care in America do, indeed, confirm that costs and access are profound difficulties.

The costs of health care have been rising over the past three decades at more than twice the rate of inflation. In 1992, Americans spent over $836 billion for health care—more than $3,000 per capita. It is estimated that national health spending for 1994 will exceed $1 trillion. Health costs consumed more than 14 percent of the Gross Domestic Product (GDP) in 1992, and, unless we find some way to control costs, that figure will be a staggering 19–20 percent by the turn of the century.

No single explanation accounts for this steady rise in costs. Various factors—medical, technological, cultural, organizational, and financial—are responsible. Medical education emphasizes reliance on tests over the development of clinical judgment; much of medical care is technologically intensive, both inside and outside the hospital. Patients are better educated, have higher expectations, and require more reassurance than at any time in the past. An aging population has more chronic diseases and more disability and requires more hospital care. Despite recent financing reforms and the enthusiasm for managed care, medical charges are still incurred and physicians continue to be compensated in ways that minimize incentives for cost consciousness among both patients and physicians. The pro-competition initiatives of the past decade have been largely ineffective. Health economists now routinely speak of costs as out of control.

Despite huge expenditures, however, there are major barriers, both financial and geographic, to health care in the United States. The poor, nonwhite, and those who live in urban ghettos and remote rural areas are in the poorest health and receive the fewest benefits. Medicaid covers less than half the poor nationally, while Medicare covers only about half of the health expenses of the elderly. At any given time, more than 37 million Americans are completely uninsured, and an equal number have inadequate insurance, meaning they would be financially ruined by a major illness or extended hospital stay. Both lack of insurance and underinsurance restrict access to health care, especially for low-income persons. The lower one's income, the greater the access problem. For example, while the top-earning 10 percent of the population spend less than 2 percent of their income on out-of-pocket medical expenses, the lowest-paid 10 percent spend, on average, 14 percent of their total income. The health care system is least available and most costly for those who need it most.

These well-known figures about the twin problems of cost and access are deeply troubling. But I will argue that the focus on these issues as the core difficulties is misplaced, and the wisdom about them is only conventional.

The fundamental problem of the U.S. health care system is neither runaway costs nor inequitable access, but lack of purpose. We simply have not decided what end, or purpose, we want to achieve in health care. At least, we have not decided with enough political conviction to enact a system that addresses this purpose in a concerted way. We have no *national* health policy. The patchwork quilt of programs we have cobbled together—for the elderly, for certain segments of the poor, for persons with specific diseases, for Native Americans, for veterans, and so on—is vivid testimony to an absence of purpose. That the current melange of programs, many created in response to crisis, works inefficiently and inequitably should come as no surprise. It was not a conscious design but a creature of incremental growth whose overall aim has never been articulated, much less publicly debated. This question of purpose is fundamentally an ethical question, not one of economics or organization.

The aim of this volume is to make the case that the question of purpose is basically one of moral and political values. I do not advocate here for one particular approach to financing and organization over others. There are no arguments in this volume for a single-payer, Canadian-style approach, or for managed competition, or for a federalist approach in which states are able to experiment within broad national standards. My aim is to infuse the debate about form and financing with the leavening of ethical analysis. Questions of reform should be seen as ethical choices, as political options for what sort of society we seek to have, and not primarily as issues of economic or organizational adjustments. Failure to see the essentially ethical and political nature of the debate will not only impoverish the rhetoric of reform; it will make it less likely that any reform we do enact will last. Health care reforms must be comprehensible morally and not just economically. Health policy must engage us in terms of common civic purpose, not only as individual consumers of health services.

I have in this work a more specific focus on universal coverage. In September 1993, President Clinton introduced the full details of his plan for health care reform, which is entitled "The Health Security Act of 1993." This plan proposes to control costs through managed competition and to provide universal coverage by 1998. While I heartily concur with the aim of ensuring coverage for everyone, I am less confident in the plan's optimistic assumptions about cost control through a more carefully managed and regulated market. If the Clinton plan, or something like it is enacted, it will take several years to implement, and the temptation to trade away universal coverage to satisfy the demands of one of the many powerful interest groups will be strong. Moreover, if the financing mechanisms do not succeed in reining in the escalation of expenses, there will be enormous pressure to abandon universal coverage in order to reduce costs. Therefore, it is essential that the American public—especially those who are well insured—have a sound understanding of why universal coverage is essential. That understanding is what this book seeks to provide.

Early in 1994 the most widely repeated prediction about health care reform was that some reform measures might be enacted in the near future but that mandatory universal coverage would not be included in these measures. This prediction is reflected in the provisions of several reform bills before Congress, which call for expanded access to be paid for by future savings or which require employers simply to offer insurance. I use the term *universal coverage* in this volume to refer to mandated coverage for everyone. A system of universal coverage means that no one is excluded. I will argue that universal coverage cannot be an aspiration deferred to better economic times, or a token gesture offered to those who are already priced out of health insurance.

Chapter 1, "Rationing and the Purpose of a Health Care System," sorts out various meanings of the term *rationing* and the assumptions these meanings bring to the discussion. The question, I will argue, is not whether health care must be rationed but how to do so fairly. The confused discussion about rationing has obscured the more important question of the purpose and aims of a health care system. I examine just how this occurs by questioning recent proposals to ration by age.

Chapter 2, "Defining a Purpose: Security and Solidarity," proposes two fundamental goals for the U.S. health care system: personal security and social solidarity. Better medical care and improved health are discussed as important particular aims, but they are rejected as overall goals. The purpose of the system, I argue, must be conceived in ethical and political terms; it transcends the peculiar aims of any of the actors, including health care providers. Theories of justice are employed near the end of the chapter as intellectual aids to clarify and sharpen perceptions of purpose, but not to set prior moral requirements for what can count as a just system.

Chapter 3, "Self-Interest and Security: A Humean Contract for Health Care," draws upon the ethical and political philosophy of David Hume to show how the goals of security and solidarity are linked. These goals are best understood as natural outgrowths of enlightened self-interest, rather than as expressions of benevolence or as communitarian virtues. My remarks here are addressed to the well-insured and what will motivate them to embrace a system of care that includes everyone.

Chapter 4, "Affinity and Solidarity: Getting from I to We," is a rebuttal of moral and social atomism. Atomism has a long and distinguished philosophical history, and it is a pervasive presence in contemporary American culture. The view of persons as discrete and self-contained units who engage in social cooperation for instrumental reasons of convenience warps the sense of self-interest that forms the argument in Chapter 3. It is impossible to move from an atomistic I to a We of genuine sociality, with the potential for solidarity. Dispelling the myth of atomism is essential for self-interest to be seen for what it is. Hume and Adam Smith (and their conceptions of sympathy) are used to explicate the native social affinity that aids benevolent tendencies and helps to sustain solidarity.

Chapter 5, "Rights and Responsibilities: Health Care Goals and Moral Coherence," argues for a right to health care as the best idiom we have to express the goals of security and solidarity. Here I am particularly concerned to make the limits to such a right morally coherent by specifying just what sort of responsibility this right entails. I argue for a Response Model over a Good Behavior Model.

While the Clinton Administration's proposals for reform (and all others I have seen) stress responsibility in terms of paying for one's care and in terms of choosing a healthy life-style, I argue that the central responsibility is for prudent use of a limited resource. Finally, I argue that patients *and* physicians should be thought of as citizens. Affirming the status of citizenship for consumers and providers both accords with medical-ethical traditions and gives a needed civic context to decisions about the judicious use of health care resources.

CHAPTER ONE

Rationing and the Purpose

of a Health Care System

The current debate over rationing health care is marked by ambiguity and confusion. Some observers argue that rationing is not inevitable and that proposals to ration are premature or even dangerous. Others claim we have been rationing all along and that the need for restrictions on health care spending will only increase. It is not always clear, however, that both sides are talking about the same thing.

Rationing as a Term of Moral Indictment

Rationing may be defined as equitable sharing of scarce goods according to a central plan. Typical cases are gasoline or food rationing in wartime. If the term is confined to this meaning, it is clear that rationing does not occur in our health care system and is not inevitable. There is no central plan for distribution of health services in the United States, and equity exists only as an ideal. Eli Ginzberg has argued that even in the face of diminishing access and escalating costs we will likely continue to improvise and make small, incremental adjustments to our current system for a long time.[1] The American desire for more medical services, together with an ingrained suspicion of government, continues to trump concerns over high costs and the embarrassing lack of access to medical services for the working poor. From this perspective rationing seems only a remote possibility.

Yet the term *rationing* has other senses and uses. Some critics of the current system have used it (and phrases like *price rationing* or *market rationing*) as a term of indictment to dramatize the way economic proclivities have usurped the concern for equality in health care.[2] Our current reliance on a market system of distribution, combined with a strong social-worth model of illness and eligibility for care, has the effect of an unfair allocation. Yet the unfairness may seem less offensive because it is the result of letting happen what is an explicit decision in other societies. Other societies ration explicitly, whereas the United States rations implicitly; others ration largely by need, while in America rationing is achieved indirectly by our reliance on a pricing system and on programs aimed at special groups, such as the elderly, veterans, or those with certain diseases. Each society sets priorities and makes decisions about which health care demands to meet. We do this also, but we don't usually call it rationing because to do so would imply limits and finite resources. American culture is ideologically committed to expanded opportunity, progress, and abundance. These cultural traits do not dispose us to contemplate shortages, limits, and hard decisions. It's easier to blame the uninsured for their lack of insurance or their ill health than to examine the structural components of a system that leaves 37 million persons uninsured and many more underserved. Examining the structural components and overall purposes of a health care system, investigating its operational logic, assessing its consequences, and debating its purpose would, after all, suggest responsibility for it.

Unfortunately, it is not clear that as a society we are ready either to acknowledge limits or to claim responsibility for how the health care system functions. So far we have conceived responsibility as largely a concern for individuals, and we therefore tend to see those services that are provided to the uninsured as "gifts" or as the bounty of our largesse.

My use of the term *rationing* to describe one facet of the current U.S. system is calculated to make an essential point.[3] This point is that allocation by price *is* a rationing scheme—one which we have largely accepted in health care as an extension of basic economic assumptions, and one which largely absolves any particular persons of responsibility for the results. Since no one actually decided to exclude the poor (as it is their lack of money and insurance, not our actions, that excludes them), no one is to blame for their exclusion.

The difficulties we have in allocating health care resources in the United States are not just quandaries about how best to distribute our resources. They are difficulties of how to *think* about our situation. One error is the idea that market forces create efficiency and restrain costs in health care. While this may be true in other sectors of the economy, it has not been true for health care. Health care costs have been rising at twice (or more) the rate of inflation over the past three decades, consuming a large and growing portion of state and federal budgets and compromising the balance sheets of corporations and the budgets of families. Obviously the higher the costs of health care, the greater the burden of those paying the bills and the fewer the number of persons who can afford the services. Rising costs have the effect of creating larger pockets of uninsured citizens. This much is obvious.

What may not be so obvious is how market forces also increase the demand for health care. The purpose of markets is not just to meet demands but to *create* demands. Markets, by definition, have no predetermined limits; it is the nature of markets to expand by creating effective demands.[4] In health care, demands are transformed by their cultural significance into needs, that is, into something more profound than a consumer desire. Moreover, in health care, our needs seem to be insatiable. Even though we have better health status than any previous generation, we worry more about our health and spend more psychic energy and monetary resources to maintain or improve it than any of our predecessors.[5] This cultural irony of being preoccupied with health while we enjoy generally good health, together with the large-scale commodification of health services, has the effect of increasing rather than reducing health care costs. While market forces may enhance efficiency in the distribution of some goods and services, in health care they drive up costs and exacerbate the problems of access. Both effects increase the numbers of citizens who are medically indigent.

Because the net effect of market forces is to create needs for those who can pay while denying access to those who cannot, I have referred to our current practices as market rationing or price rationing, to highlight both the presence of a tacit allocation policy and the role of market forces in that policy. Yet the use of terms is only a means to an end. The end, or purpose, in the use of these terms is to spur recognition and awareness of at least one of the reasons why such a disparate and inequitable system of health care allocation persists in an affluent, democratic society.

Rationing as a Term of Economic Remedy

Over the past few years the term *rationing* is increasingly being used not as an ethical critique but as a policy initiative. The term functions not to interpret and question current practices but to suggest a remedy for escalating costs. The problem it addresses is not fairness but cost containment.

It is this scenario that Arnold Relman has in mind when, in his recent editorials, he argues that rationing is not only unnecessary but impractical—it would not work. Relman believes that the elimination of waste at all levels of medical practice would yield enough funds to meet the needs of the underserved. "If physicians work in good faith with government to devise better ways to deliver health services, there is realistic hope for an affordable system that will guarantee access to an acceptable standard of care for all Americans, without resorting to rationing of any kind."[6] Wholesale reform would be necessary to make any rationing system feasible, and if the wholesale reforms were undertaken, rationing would not be needed.[7]

Relman's position is well argued and his views are widely held. Explicit policies of rationing can become an excuse for indifference to the health needs of the poor and result in an acceptance of discriminatory policies under the rubric of cost constraints. Rationing, seen as a solution, would make it the standard of practice to deny persons care that they need. The problem with rationing as a remedy is, then, that it accepts current wasteful practices as fixed and ignores the need for basic reforms in efficiency. It threatens to legitimate inadequate care under the aegis of restraints that may not be necessary.

An additional problem Relman does not discuss is the way embracing an explicit policy of rationing, as an economic remedy, can dissuade us from asking basic questions about the social purposes of medicine and health care. If we are to reform the economic incentives of the system, as Relman wants, we must also ask why we need an organized system of health care at all. What goals should the system serve? Only after we have answered this question can we devise financing schemes to meet those goals. Financing schemes and incentive systems are, after all, only means to an end. The prior question is: What sort of health care system do we want?

Relman's arguments against rationing (as a solution) are, therefore, to be applauded. Fundamental financing and administrative reforms are needed. Moreover, rationing could easily become, in the present climate, just another quick fix that fails to engage the basic question of purpose. In all these ways, the critique of rationing (as a solution) is welcome. Yet a nagging problem persists.

The problem is that arguments against explicit policies of rationing are sometimes coupled with an assumption that there need be no concern for limiting health care services. The idea that rationing is wrong because premature or unworkable, or morally wrong because discriminatory, is sometimes supplemented with a conviction that the entire concern with allocation is wrongheaded. The argument goes something like this. Who says 14 percent, or 17 percent, or even 20 percent of our gross domestic product is too much to spend on health care? When health care is weighed against other, more dubious, uses of our personal and national resources, it seems well worth the costs. Why single out health care for curtailment when tobacco subsidies (pick your favorite funding folly) go untouched?[8]

There is an important point to be made by asking this question. What will count as too much for health services will ultimately be a social and political decision. There is no natural limit to health, for health is as much cultural as biological, and there is no natural limit on the amount of resources that could be spent seeking health. Nevertheless, many believe we are approaching or have surpassed the socially appropriate limits, for there are very real social trade-offs involved in elevating health care over education, defense, or urban renewal. Lester Thurow puts it this way: "Every dollar spent on health care is a dollar that cannot be spent on something else. No set of expenditures can rise faster than the gross national product forever."[9] Thurow's views take on greater significance when international comparisons are made. In spite of the fact that we spend a larger percentage of our national wealth on health care than other nations, our health statistics lag behind. America seems to be the "odd man out" among industrialized nations when it comes to a comparison in health care budgets.[10]

Despite our disdain for thinking about limits to health care, no society has figured out how to avoid setting limits in some way. No society has devised a way to meet all the health needs of its population. Even a health care system with a parsimonious notion of need, one not inflated by utopian expectations or driven by market forces, or a system that curtailed all incentives for waste could not possibly meet all the health care needs of the population. In health care, needs will always outstrip resources. This is not just a result of perverse economic forces or wasteful practices. It is a result of how much weight is placed on health services, how pervasively important health care is for our sense (and our true state) of well-being. The idea that making technical adjustments, or even fundamentally reforming the system, will allow us to ignore the problem of setting limits is wishful thinking. Every society must decide which and whose needs to meet. The ethical question is how to decide fairly.

When rationing policies are touted as a solution to the problem of escalating costs, then, we have good reason to avoid them. Rationing practices that take the current inequities for granted and fail to call for more fundamental reforms are troubling. Those that single out vulnerable populations, as the Oregon proposals do, raise even more fundamental problems. Yet critiques that continue to assume a limitless supply or privilege health care in relation to other social needs are simply unrealistic. We can continue to be critical of the plans in Oregon, or other rationing systems, and yet still conclude that, given the options, these proposals may be the lesser of the evils open to us.[11] This conclusion is, however, unavailable to those who predicate their rejection of rationing on the assumption of limitless possibilities. Despite the problems associated with them, some explicit rationing proposals are still preferable to the tacit and irresponsible rationing practices we now have. Every rationing plan will have to be judged on its own merits, and every rationing proposal will have to be examined for its assumptions and biases. Every rationing plan will need to be balanced against current practices and not simply against the vision of an ideal system that provides everything for everyone. Whether or not we call our current practices "rationing," they effectively and systematically deny adequate care to a substantial portion of the population.

The Prior Question of Purpose

Getting clear about rationing is important, because the discussion about it has obscured an even more important question. The talk about whether we do ration implicitly, or must ration explicitly in the future, has overshadowed any consideration of purpose. What do we seek to achieve in health care? What are our goals? This is the fundamental question. Without clarity of purpose any reforms are pointless, for it will be impossible to measure success or failure. At least part of the confusion about rationing is attributable to ambiguity of purpose.

One way to understand the aims of the existing system is to take a reading from current practices. Following this method reveals two aims. The first, and perhaps the strongest, is protecting the prerogatives of physicians. Despite the fact that a large portion of the costs of medical education and almost 50 percent of total physician fees for patient care are paid from public revenues, physicians remain largely free from public accountability for the use of their skills. There are no constraints on the specialty a physician may choose (except those imposed by physicians themselves), no limits on the geographic region in which physicians may practice, and no effective restrictions on the way physicians may screen their patients and serve whomever they choose. In addition, physicians work without serious competitors and in environments designed for their convenience and largely under their control. The current system clearly protects and rewards physicians.

A second and increasingly prominent aim to be discerned from current arrangements is the protection of private markets for health insurance. For more than thirty years the federal government has intervened in health care largely to insure persons whom private insurers did not want—veterans, the elderly, the poor, and more recently persons whose diseases make them "undesirable," such as those with end-stage renal disease and HIV infection. The protection of insurers from "bad risks," underwritten by the belief that a private market for health care is workable if properly adjusted or regulated, is not just a part of the system, but one of its goals. In the belief system supporting that goal, the inability of pro-competition reforms to control costs or increase access during the past decade is explained away in terms of too little or the wrong kind of competition. The current enthusiasm for "managed competition" is testimony of the durability of this belief.

Arguments for other system goals might also be made, such as progress in biomedical research or improved health, but these are secondary. There is no close correlation between how a health care system is run and medical progress, and it would be hard to argue that the U.S. system of health care delivery is somehow more conducive to scientific advances than the systems of other countries. Improvements in health status, judging from the historical record, are more likely to come from improved living conditions and life-style changes, rather than either medical research or any particular mode of health care delivery.

But what of meeting health care needs? Surely it must be the goal of any health care system to meet needs, to cure illness when feasible and alleviate suffering when it is not. I believe an impartial observer of American health care would be hard pressed to discern this as a primary purpose of the current system. The current system does, to be sure, meet needs. The ill are frequently helped, if not always cured, and American medical-technological prowess—we are repeatedly reminded—is the envy of the world. Still, I believe that a fair conclusion is not that health care needs are met but that the health care needs *of some* are met. The uninsured receive fewer health services than the insured in both ambulatory and inpatient settings.[12] Assuming that these health services are not optional frills, the fair conclusion is that meeting needs is less important than protecting the professional prerogatives of physicians and the market prerogatives of insurers and others with vested interests. Meeting health care needs appears to be a by-product of the system, or at best a primary goal for only a select portion of the population.

Equity, I argue, would not even make the list of purposes or goals of the current system. Equity is often discussed, and it is widely embraced as a good, but there is no evidence that equitable access to care is a serious goal of our current arrangements. There is, of course, a public and professional commitment to equity once the patient is inside the hospital, or under a physician's care. But there is no strong mechanism for assuring equity of passage *into* the system; there is no equality of opportunity for becoming a patient. Medical-ethical codes, at least American twentieth-century codes, are very clear that there should be no discrimination among patients, but the same codes are equally clear that a doctor has complete freedom to select patients.

I will argue at a later point that the current goals of the U.S. health care system are wrong. But it should be noted at this point that the protection of professional prerogatives and the well-being of private insurers are not goals of the current system in any formal sense. No explicit, political decision has been made to adopt these as basic aims for which citizens would be willing to expend tax dollars. There is no regular, sustained political debate about these items. They are simply the aims of two of the most powerful players in health care. Yet the goals of providers are not the same as the overall purpose any organized system of health care would seek to achieve. To assume that they are gets the priorities backwards. Providers and insurers will, of course, work to achieve their specific purposes, and these purposes must not be inconsistent with the larger aims of a system—but they are not identical. In the absence of any overall goals, however, the separate and specific functions of the most powerful players tend to fill in the gaps and become identified—both in the popular mind and in the minds of the players themselves—as natural or self-evident goals of the entire system. Only when overall goals are clearly articulated can the aims and actions of the particular players be assessed. So in the real sense, any ethical analysis of the U.S. health care system can go no further until it is determined what is worth doing, what purposes should command our allegiance. Short of that determination of values, there is no benchmark against which to measure the actions of insurers, physicians, patients, or any of the other participants.

My chief point in this chapter is that the usual rhetoric of equity, fairness in access, cost containment, and meeting the needs of the population is not confirmed by what we see around us. As it stands, we are largely distracted from the debate about purpose by this high-minded rhetoric, and by the current confused discussion of rationing. How we will choose to ration health care is important, but the prior question is what goals we will seek to achieve through rationing.

To ask about purpose is to ask an ethical and political question. We will find the answer only by weighing the values of alternative systems in an open political process and by probing our moral convictions and our political will, not by devising new economic adjustments. Each economic and organizational reform must be judged by the extent to which it achieves the goals we seek. Ten years ago economist Lester Thurow said "Health costs are being treated as if they were largely an economic problem, but they are not. To be solved, they have to be treated as an ethical problem."[13] The chief issue in health care reform is not finding the right mix of economic adjustments, it is finding our moral and political compass.

Age-Rationing Proposals: A Case in Point

I have argued thus far that the debate about rationing is often confused and unproductive because it proceeds from unrealistic assumptions. I have also suggested that the focus on rationing draws attention away from the central issue in health policy—the question of its aim or purpose. I now want to illustrate this problem by reviewing arguments about rationing medical services by age of the patient. I will trace here the main lines of arguments of the two most influential books on this topic, Norman Daniels's *Am I My Parents' Keeper?* and Daniel Callahan's *Setting Limits: Medical Goals in an Aging Society*. Both these works are important for the development of sound health policy, but I will argue that they exhibit an additional and more important lesson than their specific policy implications for the aged. Their deeper value is in demonstrating—without necessarily intending to do so—that age-rationing cannot be entertained in the current anchorless and unprioritized set of arrangements we now have in health care.

For both Daniels and Callahan, the overriding assumption animating their analyses is the combination of scarce health care resources and near-infinite needs. Daniels begins *Am I My Par-*

ents' Keeper? with a description of the conflict over resources between young and old. Callahan constantly reminds his readers that we are on the front end of a social and medical avalanche of needs from a fast-growing elderly population. The explicit agenda motivating both books is the enormity of resources required to meet the health care needs of the elderly and whether expending such resources is fair. Is there a morally licit way to ration health care by age? For both Daniels and Callahan, the answer is a highly qualified yes, but their ways of reaching this response are very different.

Daniels and the Prudential Lifespan Account

Daniels claims that most age-rationing schemes are divisive. They tend to pit the young against the old and bespeak an adversarial framework for communication between the two groups. It is this framework that informs the rhetoric and the activities of several lobbying groups, such as the American Association of Retired Persons and Americans for Generational Equity. Within such a framework, all suggestions for transferring some resources away from the elderly toward younger groups, or vice versa, will seem discriminatory. Such transfers will inevitably seem age biased. Daniels calls this way of rendering the issues a synchronic, or slice-of-life, approach. It focuses on "age groups" at a single instant in time.

Daniels argues, by contrast, that "justice between age groups . . . is a problem best solved if we stop thinking of the old and the young as distinct groups."[14] In fact we all age; the young will eventually be the old. The task is not, therefore, one of justice between groups, not an adversarial contest of "us" versus "them," but a question of what health care resources should be available for each stage of our lives. This approach is diachronic; it conceives of persons not as representatives of their current age group but as members of a birth cohort whose needs across an entire lifespan must be considered. Only by shedding our obsession with competition for resources, Daniels claims, can we see the merits of the lifespan approach.

The question, now reformulated, is, "How would rational agents design institutions to prudently allocate fair shares of basic social goods over their lifespan?"[15] The response Daniels gives is the "Prudential Lifespan Account." It draws heavily upon the Rawlsian commitments to egalitarianism and the features of the social contract associated with the "original position." The application of these features of John Rawls's philosophy to health care issues had previously been argued in detail by Daniels.[16] The important feature of the Prudential Lifespan Account is that it offers a way to contemplate rationing by age that would not be age biased.

Daniels sums it up as follows:

> Specifically, our health-care rights might give us legitimate claims to services at one stage of our life but not at another. This may happen because meeting certain needs is more important at one stage of life than at another, or it may happen because life as a whole will be better if resources are rationed by age. The inequalities in entitlements held by different age groups do not, however, mean that people are being treated unequally, at least over the course of their lives, as I pointed out earlier. Over the lifespan, our rights to health care will be *equal* rights, even if those equal rights yield unequal entitlements at different points in the life span.[17]

In Daniels's scheme, age-rationing could be part of a larger commitment to a fair equality of opportunity. When we are young, we would equitably receive resources to assist us, with the understanding that as we age, relatively fewer resources would be expended so that the next generation may receive the same benefits we received in our youth. So what looks unfair from a slice-of-life perspective seems egalitarian from an over-a-lifetime view.

Daniels's proposal is an intriguing one and it has real merit. But as he himself acknowledges, it will make sense only within a larger social system that itself is cohesive and just. Unfortunately, our current social and political norms encourage just the opposite. The American body politic is no unified body at all but a collection of separate and largely self-interested interest groups, each lobbying fiercely for its cause and answerable only to its own constituency. In such a system, each individual or interest group is trapped inside its own slice of life, missing out on the benefits of an over-a-lifetime perspective, much less an intergenerational view.

Daniels's chief objective in *Am I My Parents' Keeper?* is to "offer a unifying vision,"[18] and in this he succeeds admirably at one level and falls short at another. He succeeds in demonstrating a nonconflictual theoretical framework for resolving allocation disputes among competing groups. His analysis is less than fully convincing because his theoretical framework is just that—not concrete, particularized, or historically nuanced enough to remedy the current practice of competition for resources. The power his vision has to command us is an intellectual power, and not yet an experientially derived power grounded in concrete recognition and lived circumstance. I will return to this criticism in Chapter 3, in reference to Hume and Rawls.

Callahan and the Natural Lifespan

A very different and more explicit argument for age-rationing is presented by Daniel Callahan. Callahan couches his argument in a sense of finitude about human life and in a redefinition of the goals of medicine. He argues that medicine should help people achieve a natural lifespan (which he defines biographically, but which generally lasts through the late seventies or early eighties) and, beyond that, it should seek to relieve suffering but not necessarily to extend life. For those who achieve a natural lifespan, treatments such as long-term mechanical ventilation and artificial resuscitation are to be avoided.

Initially, one may be tempted to see Callahan's thesis as another version of crude utilitarian thinking in health care allocation. In such a view, the old deserve less than the young because they have fewer productive years to be salvaged. This is a future-earnings, or human-capital, approach. Age is not, of course, a perfect predictor of utility, but it is on the aggregate a predictor. If we concede that interventions are less likely to be economically beneficial with the elderly and generally that the likelihood of benefit decreases with age, then treating the elderly the same as other age groups is wasteful.

This wrong-headed reading of Callahan is worth noting here because it has been cited several times in national forums. Because he has spoken forthrightly, Callahan seems especially vulnerable to vilification as a nihilist advocating passive euthanasia for the elderly on utilitarian grounds. Those who make such charges against Callahan should not be complimented as having *mis*read him, for anyone who believes that this is his position cannot have read *Setting Limits* at all. Callahan's real argument rests on two major claims, one about the ends of medicine and the other about the meaning of old age.

The aim of medicine, Callahan contends, is basically to restore health. It is not to achieve happiness, virtue, good citizenship, or even to extend or prolong life. Medicine aims, of course, to forestall premature death, but the idea of prolonging life simply to extend it temporally, to conquer death, or to arrest the aging process is untenable. It is a false goal because impossible, and the efforts to achieve it make medicine forsake its true mission.

The second major claim in Callahan's argument is his contention that a recognition of limits will benefit the elderly. Callahan claims not that the elderly do prefer a system with limits but that they ought to prefer it, because "the meaning and significance of life for the elderly themselves is best founded on a sense of limits to health care. Even if we had unlimited resources, we would still be wise to establish boundaries."[19] Callahan avoids the utilitarian, efficiency, and cost-effectiveness arguments for age-rationing. He argues rather from different norms. He rightly claims we have been held captive to a technologically driven assessment of needs that has resulted in neglect of the true social needs of the elderly. The true needs (what the elderly ought to want and what we ought to provide) are (1) as much independence as possible, (2) freedom from fear of impoverishment and other burdens of ill health, and (3) assistance to be "physically and emotionally positioned to seek whatever meaning and significance can be found in old age."[20]

Clearly, what is afoot here is a redefinition of key terms, some of which Callahan displays for the reader and some of which remain implicit. Among the explicated terms are *natural lifespan* (measured in both biographical and biological terms), *tolerable death* (what occurs at the end of a natural lifespan), and *need* (a socially defined requirement, not a function of technological capacity). What remain tacit and undefined are terms like *nature* (including *human nature*), various meanings of *old age,* and the deep implications of *stewardship* of resources grounded in intergenerational fidelities. There is, however, a strong sense throughout that some variation of traditional Christian theological renderings of these terms would probably do quite well as definitions for Callahan's purposes.

I do not cite this lack of explicitness in order to criticize Callahan. He has done an admirable job presenting a controversial and courageous thesis in a brief, accessible volume. Explications of the sort philosophers hanker after would have doubled the size of the book. Rather, I cite these terms and their axial position in his thesis to raise a query about the extent to which readers share Callahan's framework. Are these terms and their implications available, comprehensible, or morally forceful only inside a religious community or can they work, roughly, to explicate an ethic for a decidedly pluralistic social order (or disorder)? The verdict is, perhaps, still out, at least for health care. What is noteworthy about Callahan's effort is that his appeal is not to individuals in their posture as prudent calculators of personal gain. Rather, he invokes a vision of the social good in which individuals will be at least partially governed in their choices for medical care and policies by an ethic that transcends private interests. So while Daniels is concerned to show how private individuals might validly choose for public benefit out of their own self-interest, Callahan wants to show how a public and social good is the context for any private choice that could count as virtuous. His insistence that prudence and limits in health care will be better for the elderly themselves points to a notion of private or personal good not tethered to survival but to the intrinsic worth of life in a community. He calls upon readers to use an idiom that does not begin from an assumption that private good can be defined independently, as a free-standing entity. Private and individual goods for Callahan are inseparable from public and social life.

The limiting force for Callahan's thesis—as he acknowledges—is the lack of a larger moral and political context. Restricting the life-extending health care of the elderly in the absence of meeting their larger social needs and in the absence of a social network that supports prudence in all sectors of health policy would be pernicious. Or, to put it differently, why should we insist that the needs of the elderly be redefined if we (the nonelderly) are unwilling (or unable) to redefine our own? Without more generally accepted prudential policies, the elderly would not benefit at all; they would simply lose one set of services without gaining other (more fitting) ones. In the absence of larger social changes, the elderly would be foolish to go along.

Avoiding Piecemeal Reforms

The proposals of both Daniels and Callahan have proved to be controversial. Criticism of Callahan's suggestion of a specific age for a natural lifespan has overshadowed his more important points. Daniels's concerns are more theoretical and are calculated to show that a properly conceived age-rationing scheme need not be discriminatory. My task here is not to adjudicate among these authors and their critics but to point to the inevitable difficulties when specific programs are recommended in the absence of coherent health policy.

Daniels notes that his proposals rely on at least two "ideal" theoretical features. First, prudent choosers are asked to make choices "on the assumption that there is already compliance with other, more general principles of distributive justice." Second, the prudent deliberators assume that there will be general compliance with the principles of distribution they choose.[21] Yet these conditions are not just "ideal" in the theoretical sense. They are unrealistic in the political sense. Indeed, Daniels later gives a penetrating account of the enormous difficulties in making any such ideal assumptions work in his discussion of how difficult it is for U.S. physicians to say "no" to patients, concluding that "the system as a whole is not governed by a principle of distributive justice . . . our system is not closed under constraints of justice."[22]

Callahan, in a similar vein, is acutely aware that the social and political conditions that would support his age-rationing proposals are not present in late-twentieth-century America. Indeed, his subsequent book, *What Kind of Life*, is partially devoted to raising larger questions that would provide the necessary context for *Setting Limits*.[23]

I have sympathy for Callahan's views, and what I propose in this volume is in some ways a continuation of his work—yet with an important difference. Callahan is exquisitely clear about the hazards of making our personal aspirations for better health or greater longevity the driving force of a health care system. He is equally lucid about the problems that ensue if health care is dominated by a zeal for medical progress through technology. Indeed, the subtitle of *What Kind of Life* is *The Limits of Medical Progress*. The key difference is that Callahan's focus is on the relative value of health in personal and social life, whereas my concern is to see medical services and health policy as part of social policy.

If health care is ever to be reformed it will be because we finally address the issue as the problem of what social aims are to be pursued. By contrast, the usual way of discussing reform is to begin with a minute analysis of the problems in one specific segment of health care organization, financing, or delivery or of the values involved, such as the amount of care provided to the aged, the reimbursement of physicians, the distribution of doctors, or the number of procedures or hospital days per capita. Yet none of the information coming from these sophisticated studies, by itself, has any necessary bearing on what a health care system ought to be doing. At best they are partial solutions in some system yet to be clearly articulated, and at worst irrelevant. No recommendation makes sense in the absence of an answer to the prior question of purpose.

Health policy must stand on its own feet as a social and political choice. There is no other beginning point. To focus the issue in terms of cost problems, insurance problems, access problems, and so on in the usual litany is to place the cart before the horse. The result is to make the purpose and goals of the health care system no more than the sum of adjustments to these particular practices. Depending on the predilections of the experts, some aspect of the current arrangements is usually privileged, just as the Clinton Administration proposals now seem to privilege the place of management through competition. This confuses ends and means. Better management through competition might provide adjustments to current practices, but it will not qualify as health care system reform unless it is in the clear service of explicit goals.

In *What Kind of Life* Callahan argues that health care should be seen as a means to the other goals we wish to achieve in life, not as an end in itself. In this volume I am arguing that we must conceive of the health care system as having its own goals, not as a euphemism for practices of compensating doctors or providing insurance coverage. A health care system must stand for something on its own. It should, of course, shape practices in matters like cost, access, eligibility, and the like, but it must also be guided by explicit priorities about the uses of social resources broadly conceived, and it must address issues of the common weal.

I will discuss definitions of purpose in detail in the chapter to follow. For now I want to underline the central point that justifies the mode of approach I am taking. However elegant and appealing they are, proposals to ration services by age, or by any other criteria, are premature and potentially distracting. The root issue is what kind of health care system we want, not what particular services we think the elderly should have. Outside this larger context, age-rationing proposals are just another gimmick in the long line of improvisations we have devised to "fix" immediate problems. Going about health care reform in this piecemeal fashion is no more likely to be effective than our attempts to control costs by regulating physician fees on a procedure-by-procedure basis.

CHAPTER TWO

Defining a Purpose:

Security and Solidarity

To inquire about the purpose of a health care system is to ask what fundamental goals could be used to explain why the system should be as it is. If we are to succeed in this inquiry we must avoid thinking in too narrow or too grandiose a fashion.

In the previous chapter I argued that the debates about rationing often go nowhere because the various understandings of this term, and the proposals for specific programs, lack a common context. These are instances of thinking that is too narrow; discussion is hampered by the focus on specifics in the absence of agreement on the larger issues. Other examples are ready at hand. For instance, goals for the health care system could be set by reference to the aspirations of the Human Genome Initiative. This research program is intended to supply vast amounts of genetic information and possibly genetic therapies—at a cost in dollars and a potential loss in privacy yet to be reckoned—and it is not unreasonable to think of these objectives as candidates to fill the current void in health care goals. There are already those who are worried about a "geneticization" of medicine and health care, with an accompanying neglect of the social causes of diseases.[1] Indeed, defining health system goals primarily through scientific medical achievements (or aspirations) is perhaps the greatest temptation currently leading us to an overly narrow conception of purpose.

The opposite problem is a tendency toward grandiosity. This is the assumption (or hope) that a single purpose could be universally affirmed for the entire system and that new goals would be embraced and pursued unambiguously. This ideal would fit nicely with American nostalgia for a return to the simplicity of an organic community, or Gemeinschaft. Even a culture as self-conscious about pluralism and diversity as ours harbors such longings, perhaps precisely because pluralism and diversity are seen as enduring social characteristics.

Although I hope that many will agree with the goals I discuss here in defining a purpose for health care, I cannot hope for universal assent. Nor do I offer these as anything more than provisional statements that, even if accepted, will need examination and refinement. Indeed, the wish for clear and unambiguous goals is the wish to have a purpose established independent of the political process and the give-and-take of arguments about social priorities. In fact, until recently one of the operative assumptions in the United States was that health care is so important that it need not be weighed in comparison with other social programs. What we desperately need now is a sustained debate about purpose and goals in which these comparisons can be made. My list in this chapter is intended as a beginning statement, one that will at least give us something to hold on to as we work for reform.

A final caveat concerns the approach I take here. Bioethical issues are usually examined through the lens of a theory of justice, frequently focused on the question whether a right to health care is to be affirmed or denied. For example, the recent insightful work of Charles Dougherty in *American Health Care* follows this line of inquiry, considering in turn utilitarian, egalitarian, libertarian, and contract theories and finally opting for "pluralistic foundations" combining elements of each.[2]

I will eschew this way of proceeding in part because it has been done well by others, but primarily because of the hazards it entails. To begin with theories and work one's way to rights, then to policy aims and goals, runs the risk that the requirements of theory will overdetermine the goals. If properly applied, a utilitarian theory should only tell us what a utilitarian health goal would be, in the same way that beginning with a market theory of how health care should be organized and financed will lead to some form of competition, "managed" or otherwise. Even an approach not tied to one theory but endorsing a variety of theories is hazardous. And if, as Dougherty argues, theories must be selectively used, perhaps it would be better to use them afterward, less as a point of entry and more as a way to test and deepen our prior thinking. This is the approach I will use here.

This method is more direct and empirical; it relies less on what theory directs and more on what I take to be common experiences of, and aspirations for, health care. In staying closer to the ground I do not wish to gainsay the usefulness of ethical theories (or for that matter economic theories). Theories are exceedingly useful to clarify, make consistent, test, and hopefully support what experience tells us. But theories are by definition remote from our experiences, and using them to set our goals may give them a larger place in the deliberations than is merited.

I choose this approach not because no one theory of justice enjoys universal assent. It is not a method taken up as a fallback position, or a second-best way to proceed because, for example, we are not all utilitarians, or all libertarians, about health care. Rather, this more intuitive and experiential method is needed because health goals are not theoretical products. Just the opposite assumption would be more accurate. Decisions about goals will direct our attention to those theories thought to be relevant and determine which features of these theories are most germane. It is perhaps in its favor that this mode of proceeding is more in keeping with the way most ethical decisions are actually made: decisions are usually reached first, and greater intellectual coherence and justifications are sought afterward.

Why Better Medical Care and Improved Health Are Not Goals

In this section I list my candidates for the goals of a health care system. It may be surprising to some that better medical care or improved health, to take two examples, are not listed among these goals. Their absence is not an oversight.

In the opening statement of his book *Medical Care, Medical Costs*, Rashi Fein says, "Health care policy is a part of social policy."[3] It would be easy to brush aside this statement and say, "Of course, it could hardly be otherwise." Yet I want to probe its deeper implications, which I believe are reflected in the way Fein addresses the insurance question in his book. Health care policy is a part of social policy in the sense that it is primarily a matter of what sort of society we wish to have. This means that although health policy is concerned with doctors, patients, medical research, public health measures, and many other particulars involved in the delivery of care, health care policy is fundamentally about the way these things are understood. Health care policy is a matter of how these powerful players and agendas are to be ordered, and of the relative importance of health care in the larger scheme of things. Thus, contrary to expectations, a health care system should not have as its primary goal better medical care or the promotion of better health, valuable as these things are.

This may seem a bizarre claim to make, perhaps because current U.S. health care arrangements are dominated by medical, scientific, and business professionals who have used our aspirations for health as a lever to enlarge their activities. Whatever the reason, this unseasonable claim is central to my argument, and is in fact quite simple. Maximizing health, promoting well-being, discovering new therapies, and many other things we prize are the proper aims of providers, patients, researchers, and public health officials at a variety of levels. Yet when these role-specific functions become fundamental goals of a health care system, the system becomes misdirected. To be sure, a health care system should support activities that promote better health, better training for professionals, progress in research, and so on. No system can be antithetical to these activities. But, again, the system goals must be larger; they are, properly speaking, moral and political agendas. Otherwise there is no way to assess when the personal zeal for health, or the enthusiasm for scientific progress in medical research, is excessive.

The need to frame our goals in this way may be further clarified by an analogy. The U.S. military system equips its troops with the best and most effective weapons available to maintain a fighting force that is, in the accepted jargon, "second to none." Yet it is clearly understood that military aims are part of a larger system of defense, in the service of the national interests. Guns, tanks, planes, and soldiers have no purpose independent of their national purpose. Similarly, doctors, hospitals, health insurers, researchers, and all the other players cannot be left free to define for themselves whatever goals they wish, unless we decide to give up on the task of constructing a coherent health care system altogether. Whatever system we devise must order and regulate the activities and ambitions of these players, less they turn public resources to their own private ends.

By making this analogy I am not implying that the federal government needs to own and operate the means of providing health care, as in a national health service. I am rather pointing out the difference between system goals, which relate to social purposes, and the goals of particular players, who are naturally concerned with their daily, role-specific functions. Doctors cannot independently decide on the goals of a health care system any more than generals can decide, by themselves, on the defense goals of the country.

One final possible misunderstanding needs to be addressed. A great deal has been said about the growing "medicalization" of society, that is, the tendency to define social, spiritual, legal, and other sorts of problems as diseases. More and more of life is being subject to medical therapeutics, and health professionals are being given increasing control over lives and budgets. Daniel Callahan, for example, is eloquent on this point, arguing for a parsimonious notion of needs and against a medical understanding of what are essentially social needs.[4] It may seem that my point about the fundamentally moral and political nature of health care goals will move us toward more medicalization, rather than less. This would be a mistaken interpretation.

I agree with Callahan and others that medicine cannot solve (at least by itself) many of the chronic problems of society, such as substance abuse, teenage pregnancy, homelessness, or violence, nor should it be expected to do so. But my point here is a different one. While we have expected too much of medicine in one sense, we have expected too little in another sense. We have dumped those problems we find distasteful or intractable into physicians' laps, and these expectations have been too great. But neither have we given physicians a clear social agenda within which to work, and here our expectations have been too few. It is not surprising, then, that a great number of social ills get defined in medical terms. There is no social policy to define medicine's boundaries or specify its range of responsibilities. Once a clear agenda is established, "medicalization" should be less of a problem.

Security and Solidarity

Any health care system should have two primary goals. The first is *security*, by which I mean the freedom of persons to live without fear that their basic health concerns will go unattended, and freedom from financial impoverishment when seeking or receiving care.

In any given case, treatment of any illness may or may not be effective, and a health care system can do little to change this. The effectiveness of treatments is a function of the state of the art and the skills of practitioners, and the quality of the educational system that trains providers. What a good health care system should offer, and practitioners cannot, is coverage for preventive services and for diagnosis and treatment of disease by current standards of care. This is a policy determination, not a matter of the actions of individual practitioners considered separately.

The goal of security can be stated in the negative as follows. No specific player in health care should have power to deny persons secure access to what the system offers, or to threaten them with impoverishment (or in other ways mitigate their access). We now have a system in which the most powerful figures—physicians, hospitals, insurance companies, pharmaceutical firms—have vested interests that compromise the security of many of those who seek care. The details of these arrangements are well known, and it would be tedious to enumerate them here. It should be the aim of our health care system to eliminate the conflict between the self-interest of any of these figures and the security of persons in seeking and receiving care.

The second goal is *solidarity*, which is the sense of community that emerges from acknowledgment of shared benefits and burdens. Solidarity is a feature of the health care systems in many European countries. Although many Americans might affirm solidarity as a good thing to have, few would think to include it in the basic goals a health care system should strive to achieve. Americans are often ambivalent and suspicious of communitarian ambitions, which they tend to see as infringements on freedom. Moreover, the nostalgic, utopian side of the American attraction toward community carries a bias that communities are not things to be built. In this vein of thinking, communities exist as a consequence of transcendent powers, like the church, or blood ties, or even the shared experience of a catastrophe, as many survivors of the floods of 1993 have testified.

Social solidarity in health care does not directly derive from these springs of community, though it can be related to any of them. Rather, it is grounded in understanding the value of sharing common resources, resources that are universally needed, acknowledged to be scarce, and supported by public revenues and energies. These are the rational grounds for solidarity. The affective grounds have to do with the urge to belong, to see one's own situation as like that of others, to notice and affirm affinities in the human condition. This sense of affinity is closely related to motivations of benevolence.

Security is focused on individual and personal well-being while solidarity has to do with our relationships with others. In health care these aims are complementary. Security is not attainable without solidarity, and solidarity is meaningless unless it ensures the security of each individual. The reasons for choosing these two goals will be the concern of subsequent chapters. I will argue that both self-interest and more benevolent motives should impel us to embrace these aims.

By stressing only these two aims I do not gainsay other aspects of a health care system. For example, any organized system for delivering care must be efficient, and it must be in accord with the professional values of the providers who work within it. These and other obvious prerequisites could be called goals in a secondary sense, but not in the most basic sense. Efficiency, however important, is always in the service of some other purpose. "Efficiency for what?" is always a viable question. And while a health care system cannot be inconsistent with practitioners' values or interests, satisfying these should be seen as a lubricant to the system rather than its basic aim.

In his address to Congress of September 22, 1993, introducing his plans for health care reform, President Clinton listed six goals—security, simplicity, savings, choice, quality, and responsibility. All six goals are important, but they are not equal in importance. For example, while patients clearly need some choices about providers and treatments, making choice a paramount value turns patients into customers and health services into commodities. Simplicity, to take another of the six, is usually an asset but it isn't necessarily a fundamental component of a just system. I will have more to say about responsibility in Chapter 5. Solidarity, the second of my two goals for a health care system, is not yet as politically palatable as choice or savings are, but it must become so. There can be no health care security without it.

The concrete meanings of security and solidarity were powerfully exemplified for me in the late spring of 1993. My wife and I were walking a path on the Quiraing, a mountainous ridge on the Isle of Skye, Scotland. It was unusually dry on Skye that spring, and my wife slipped on the loose stones, suffering a severe ankle fracture. Two hours later, with the help of several other hikers and the Royal Air Force mountain rescue team, we were helicoptered off the ridge to the major medical center in Inverness. Eight days later we were aboard a return flight to the United States.

The health care my wife received in Scotland was remarkable in many ways. She never received a number, nor was she ever addressed by diagnosis, but always by name, as Mrs. Churchill. The use of names is not just an act of courtesy, but a sign that patients are recognized as persons. The hospital staff was professional in every way—competent, efficient, and polite. Their morale was high and they took obvious pride in their work. The surgery was as technically competent as could be experienced anywhere in this country. During each of the seven hospital days tea was served at 10:00 A.M. and 3:00 P.M. to everyone in the ward—patients, family, visitors, and staff. In short, the care was technically competent and humane, but it also conveyed an air of conviviality and community. All this meant a great deal, but it is not my main point.

Although we were foreigners, there was never a question of treatment being delayed, abbreviated, or altered in any way. After five days I realized that no one had inquired about our insurance status, and money had never been discussed. So on the day before our scheduled departure I made arrangements to see the surgeon on morning rounds to discuss the charges. As we would be leaving soon, I explained, I wanted to inquire about his fee and how it could be paid. "Fee?" he said. "Nothing to do with me!" And he added, "Thank God." He walked away assuring me that my wife could make the trans-Atlantic flight in a cast with no problem and explaining how the cast would be split and bound to accommodate the swelling.

A nurse, overhearing this conversation, suggested I talk to the ward registrar about any fees. The ward registrar sent me to the hospital business office. Here I was told, in a tone of apology, that "Yes, there will be charges." Apparently it has been the practice to charge foreigners for medical services only since the late 1980s and the Thatcher "reforms" to the National Health Service. Even now charges are made only for those visitors from countries with no reciprocal agreement to care for U.K. travelers. The bill I was given at that time was an estimate, and we were sent the exact charges only six weeks after our return home. It consisted of two items: a flat per diem charge for the hospital and an additional charge for the use of the operating room, noted as "theatre time." The total for a one-week hospital stay and a complicated surgical procedure amounted to $3,829.

What is remarkable to me is not so much the low cost (equivalent services in the U.S. would exceed $12,000), but that costs were addressed so late in the process. Americans are accustomed to displaying their insurance cards and filling out forms prior to admission. Even emergency admissions are often punctuated by a clerk with an insurance form in hand. Before leaving the business office at Inverness I signed a form stating that I would endeavor to pay the bill we would receive upon returning home. I shook hands with the business manager and left. I recount this not as a model of hospital efficiency, but as a detail consistent with all the other patient-centered practices we encountered. At Inverness, it was never suggested that our access to care was in any way contingent upon our ability to pay. Such practices are an embodiment of security.

I spent the week in Inverness at a hotel near the hospital. The proprietors, a Scottish couple in their mid-fifties, were conscious of my predicament as a foreign traveler with an injured spouse. Late in the week, after one of my daily progress reports, the husband remarked, "Isn't our health care system a wonderful thing?" I heartily agreed. Every aspect of my wife's care had been excellent. Upon reflection what strikes me is not the quality of the services, but that these services could be referred to as part of "*our* health care system." The system belongs to the population as a whole, and it is a point of pride to most U.K. residents that it is inclusive. This is the meaning of solidarity. There is no American equivalent. I can only say, "How lucky I am to have health insurance." There is no "our" system with which to identify, no "we" of solidarity encompassing everyone.

Theories in the Service of Goals

Earlier I rejected the use of theories of justice as the primary methodological instruments in our search for purpose. The fundamental goals of a health care system, I argued, must be more concretely perceived. They should not be a function of intellectual acumen in deducing, or failing to deduce, a right to health care from theoretical requirements about fairness, freedom, or various conceptions of the good. Thus I have sought to avoid prejudicing my formulations with the commitments of contract theories, libertarianism, and other intellectual devices. Proceeding in this way does not place us in opposition to theories of justice but rather in favor of their judicious use. It now remains to show what a judicious use might be.

Since Aristotle justice has been roughly formulated as the principle of giving each person his or her due, that is, treating equals equally and unequals according to their inequalities.[5] The debates in theories of justice are largely concerned with which inequalities are relevant. Distributive justice concerns benefits and burdens and how they affect individuals, groups, or classes of people. Theories of distributive justice in health care are, therefore, ways of formulating principles or rules for the allocation of benefits and burdens so that the relevant (and only the relevant) inequalities come into play.

Using theories of distributive justice in health care is difficult for two reasons. First, there is a vast array of procedures and services that fall under the category of health care, from facelifts to inoculations, from wellness clinics to heart transplants. Second, access to health care is valued differently not only by different people but by the same person at different times. Health care may not seem important if we perceive ourselves as well, but it becomes essential if we believe we are ill. On the other hand, it has proven easier to think clearly about other goods and services. Color televisions, for example, are universally distributed by market forces, and the relevant inequality is the ability to pay. Olympic medals, by contrast, are distributed by athletic prowess, and inequality is measured by performance (not medically or chemically enhanced) while race, age, or social status are irrelevant inequalities. In most societies access to some degree of public education is offered to all, and native intelligence and social standing are considered irrelevant inequalities. Burdens are borne in proportionately equal terms through tax-based revenue systems. In each of these and many other areas, the knotty issues of distribution are generally settled, but in health care (at least in the United States) the question of what counts as a relevant inequality is contested terrain. Each society must finally settle on a method for allocating health services, though there is no reason to believe that the method chosen must be the same as that by which goods and services are generally allocated, or that the same method must be used for all health care goods and services. For example, preventive services and treatment for hypertension could be distributed in one fashion and rhinoplasty in another. It should not be expected, or demanded, that a single principle or set of principles must speak to health care as a whole.

An exhaustive, or even a representative, historical account of the many theories of justice of possible relevance to health care would be too much to attempt. I will confine myself to the major modern theories of justice, that is, to those usually cited in attempts to sort out the relevant inequalities in distribution. I will review these theories not as contributions of specific theorists, but in terms of types, giving representative thinkers for each type. My aim is not to argue for one theory over others but to suggest that each has a place in deepening our understanding of the goals for health care I have listed. The task is to discern and incorporate the insights of each while being aware of blind spots.

Egalitarianism

Egalitarian theories emphasize similarities or equalities among persons. Such theories typically embrace notions of intrinsic worth, that is, those aspects of persons which are *not* instrumental to achieving some other good but in terms of which persons are to be valued for their own sake. Egalitarian theories of health care distribution focus on the *need* for services—not money, insurance, age, or other factors, which are deemed irrelevant—as the basic criterion for allocation. Egalitarian theories are supported not only by the recognition of the equal intrinsic worth of persons but by a common human vulnerability to disease, disability, and death, by our usual inability to predict the timing or extent of our health care needs, and by the importance of health services to our dignity and self-respect as well as life and health. Michael Walzer puts it this way.

> Were medical care a luxury, these discrepancies [in access to care] would not matter much; but as soon as medical care becomes a socially recognized need, and as soon as the community invests in its provision, they matter a great deal. For then deprivation is a double loss—to one's health and to one's social standing.[6]

Many egalitarian theorists believe the best approach comes from applying the principles of John Rawls to health policy.[7] Rawls contends that inequalities in the distribution of the primary goods of a society can be tolerated only if these inequalities are to everyone's advantage. Whether health care is a primary good is a contested notion. Norman Daniels argues that equitable distribution would provide a fair "equality of opportunity" for "species-typical normal functioning."[8] Some degree of health care is clearly required for opportunity to achieve normal functioning, and the liberties and goods that accrue from normal functioning.

Egalitarians frequently speak of health care as a right. For some this is a right of equal access to all that is available. Others see this right more modestly as a right to a decent or basic minimum, with a varying list of what counts as basic.

The typical strengths of egalitarian theories are the emphases on intrinsic worth, the high ideals they hold out, and their descriptions of things humans hold (and suffer) in common. Egalitarian theories frequently resonate with those aspects of religious traditions which eschew judgments of social worth and which favor the poor and disenfranchised. However, they clash with those aspects of religious traditions which emphasize hierarchies of power and which value spiritual life over bodily health.

The weaknesses of egalitarian approaches are in part definitional and operational. What, after all, is a health care need and who should define it? Our health needs seem to expand daily and our appetite for health, at least in the United States, has yet to find a natural limit. For example, the move twenty years ago to guarantee everyone a right to treatment for end-stage renal disease has become so costly as to deprive the populace of other basic needs, both medical and nonmedical. Despite these problems, and critiques from the utilitarian and libertarian camps, it should be noted that egalitarian theories of justice provide the most fertile ground for a right to care.

Utilitarianism

Utilitarian theories reference the rightness or wrongness of actions or policies to the good or bad consequences they generate. While egalitarian theories emphasize intrinsic worth, utilitarian approaches avoid judging policies by their intentions in favor of empirical results. Right acts and policies are those which issue in the most good achieved, or the greatest net happiness for the greatest number. For some utilitarians, such as Jeremy Bentham, all kinds of happiness count, which means that the calculation of the greatest good is purely quantitative.[9] Others, such as John Stuart Mill, have developed hierarchies of happiness such that the higher pleasures, or those distinctive to human fulfillment, count for more.[10]

Utilitarianism does not endorse, as is sometimes thought, egoistic hedonism, such that only my own pleasure counts in the calculations. To the contrary, it is the well-being or happiness of all that matters, and each is to be counted neutrally and equally. If anything, utilitarian theories may actually require more disinterested judgments about our own lives than most of us are capable of.

Regarding health care policies, utilitarian approaches ask us to weigh the benefits and burdens of various policies of allocation and to be guided by the results. Would the greatest net happiness be achieved by policies that grant an entitlement to all or by policies that restrict access in some fashion? Would the greatest good be reached by dismantling redundant technological apparatus for tertiary care in favor of housing and nutritional programs? Although utilitarians do not usually advocate radical positions of change, they are theoretically open to any course that would achieve the desired end. If we were to attempt such calculations for health care, a great deal would have to be considered, for example, the happiness of those treated, the tax burdens of those who pay, the impact of discontinuing, curtailing, or expanding a program, and so on. The well-being of patients, nonpatients, physicians, and others, indeed all others, would be important. The key elements here are the absence of intrinsic or innate values that might countervail our ability to assess the outcomes and the irrelevance of motives and intentions. Goodness, in utilitarian thinking, is not a state of will or an internal motivation of the heart, but a real, measurable item in the world. Moreover, it is not just what I want, but what would be good when the well-being of all is considered.

The strengths of utilitarian approaches are numerous. The emphasis on empirical reality rather than inner motives makes for more accessible and public judgments and can serve to open discussion to a broad range of participants and possibilities. Additionally, utilitarianism, at least in its most influential forms, encourages impartiality in the sense that each person's happiness counts but no one's happiness counts more than others. Some are attracted to utilitarianism for its simplicity. Rather than a complex bevy of rules and maxims, a single principle concerning outcomes and events is offered. Finally, utilitarian schemes seem to have a natural affinity with democratic governmental practices. It is no accident that Bentham's and Mill's utilitarian philosophies have underwritten a number of social and political reforms in England in the nineteenth and twentieth centuries.

Still, the liabilities are substantial. A standard for justice which is referenced solely to outcomes must rely on the ability to predict outcomes correctly. This can be a difficult task. Others have worried that utilitarian approaches are counter-intuitive. If everyone's happiness is to be counted as equal to my own, does this mandate the most extraordinary self-sacrifice? Moreover, if everyone's happiness is to count equally, does this mean that a physician's obligations to strangers are equal to her obligations to her patients? Utilitarianism would seem to undercut some of our most deep-seated notions of loyalty and fidelity. Finally, and perhaps most importantly, does the emphasis on the greatest happiness mean that great suffering for a few can be tolerated so long as the vast majority benefit? Would this encourage neglect of some patients to achieve a greater aggregate good?

From a utilitarian perspective, whether there is a right to health care is contingent upon whether such a right would be instrumental for achieving the best overall outcome. It is, then, a question to be settled empirically, by comparative studies of the results, rather than answered on grounds of the intrinsic worth of persons or an egalitarian regard for well-being.

Libertarianism

Libertarian approaches to justice stand in stark contrast to the two previously discussed. Whereas both egalitarian and utilitarian approaches present alternative conceptions of the common good, libertarian thinking questions the independent existence of common or social goods.

Robert Nozick, with Ockhamite parsimony, states the position forcefully. Pointing out that as individuals we frequently undergo sacrifices for a greater personal good, Nozick asks:

> Why not, similarly, hold that some persons have to bear some costs that benefit other persons more, for the sake of the overall social good? But there is no *social entity* with a good that undergoes some sacrifice for its own good. There are only individual people, different individual people, with their own individual lives. Using one of these people for the benefit of others, uses him and benefits the others. Nothing more.[11]

Libertarianism, as the name suggests, values liberty, and its cardinal virtue is noninterference with others. This is not to say that other virtues—courage, loyalty, respect for others, beneficence—are not also valued, but only liberty is a *fundamental* right. The Bill of Rights of the U.S. Constitution is frequently cited as a prominent example of libertarian thinking. The rights of free speech, assembly, religious worship, and so on are seen primarily as rights to be left alone, rights not to be coerced by others, especially by government. Positive rights, rights that require obligations from others for their fulfillment, are not rights at all but claims, which can (usually) only be satisfied by violating the basic rights of others. Hence, libertarians generally believe that there is no right to health care services, since providing those services would involve coercing taxpayers to fund them and physicians to perform them. Inequities in health and health care are then seen as unfortunate, but not unfair. If the poor die from lack of services while others pay for it and survive, it may be regrettable but it is not unjust. If charitable tendencies in society prevail, and funds are donated so that doctors and hospitals can give to the poor what they need, then the donors are to be commended. But there is no duty for any individual to contribute resources to fund health care, and the poor have no claim to receive care, no right to demand it.

Libertarians place a high premium on protection of property, including financial resources. Possessions are seen as extensions of their owners. In a frequently quoted article against a right to health care, Robert Sade claims that since a physician owns his professional skills, he is entitled to do with them as he pleases. As bread belongs to the baker, to dispose of as he wishes, so medical services belong to the physician.[12] To force him to follow a fee schedule, to require him to provide services or to see patients against his wishes, is a fundamental breech of liberty.

Justice, in libertarian terms, is simply respecting the freedoms of persons and keeping hands off what they rightfully own. The idea that someone else may have a right to what one owns is frequently attributed, in libertarian thinking, to envy. Just because the poor envy the health care services of the rich does not entitle them to the same services. Rights claims, when they require redistribution of property, should be seen as nothing more than the politics of envy, so the libertarian argument often goes.

The strengths of libertarian thinking are obvious, at least to many Americans. The current U.S. health care system is basically libertarian in orientation: it distributes the goods and services of health care on the basis of purchasing power and the ownership of health insurance. Libertarian approaches dovetail with laissez-faire economics, in health care and in most other sectors of society. Although many physicians chafe under the regulations and restrictions of third-party payers and managed-care practices, these efforts at cost control are adjustments to market forces, not alternative models of justice. In addition to protecting economic freedoms, libertarianism appeals to our sense of respect for personal freedoms. This strikes a favorable chord with both patients and physicians. For patients it can mean the ability to choose one's doctor and negotiate the conditions of one's care. For physicians freedom to practice is often translated as freedom to make clinical judgments without interference and is seen, therefore, not merely as politically appropriate but as the essence of professionalism, as "good medicine." Finally, libertarianism serves as a warning about the growth and hegemony of state power, and as such it has a lasting appeal to anyone at all distrustful of concentrations of power in any form.

The weaknesses of libertarian approaches are the strengths of egalitarian and utilitarian philosophies. First, libertarianism seems blind to commonalities among people and to the degree of shared circumstances in contemporary societies. With its strident emphasis on negative freedom, the libertarian position seems better suited to individuals attempting to break away from the repressive societies of the past. It isn't clear that an ethic that protects all freedoms is the best or primary value for citizens of modern industrial democracies.

Other critics have focused on libertarianism's orientation toward property rights. Historically, it isn't always clear that current property holdings have been acquired fairly (by noncoercive means). Hence, some redistributive schemes that favor the less well-off may amount to restorative justice. Additionally, portraying physicians' knowledge and skills as private possessions for sale ignores the large contributions from public funds that train physicians, support hospitals, and subsidize payments for patient services. For example, roughly half the costs of medical training, and half the costs of medical services, are paid from public funds, rather than from the private resources of individuals.[13] This represents a substantial transfer of wealth into the hands of a few professionals who are granted, by license, a monopoly over services. A duty to serve publicly determined health needs could be seen as a reasonable "fee" for this transfer of wealth and power to physicians. Medicine could not be practiced in anything like its present form without the "coercive" hand of government subsidies and public tax support.

Finally, libertarian approaches ring true only if health is thought of as a private possession rather than a public good. A completely individualistic approach to health needs, in which concerted public and social efforts were eliminated, would result in a substantial decrease in services rendered and in the health of the population.

Using Theories to Clarify Goals

Theories of justice are important not because they will provide an air-tight case for any particular health care policy but because they help us think clearly about the goals of any policy. Each theory works from a different sense of what is important about persons, what is fair, and what constitutes a good society. No one theory has gained universal acceptance, since no one theory captures all the dimensions of fairness or all the values of persons and communities that we deem important. The best approach to health care will therefore be an eclectic and pluralistic one, an approach that seeks to use the salient aspects of each theory to help clarify our sense of what kind of health care system we want and can live with.

We know from egalitarian theories, for example, that security concerns are universal. Each person's health security is equivalent to every other person's. If there is to be a right to health care, it must be universal in scope. Yet because they cannot readily rank hierarchies of need, egalitarian theories generally do not indicate how to restrict entitlements to health care in such a way that society can feasibly satisfy them.

A utilitarian approach is helpful at precisely this point. Because it references the good solely to aggregate outcomes, utilitarianism has little or no way to appreciate the problems of personal security. But it can be very serviceable in determining what health benefits should be offered beyond the minimum package that would satisfy security concerns. In utilitarianism all therapies beyond the minimum package would have to be weighted in the interest of the greatest overall good; a health care system organized in this way would gain a common allegiance beyond that earned by a system ensuring only some people's personal security. Thus, utilitarian approaches undergird solidarity by giving allocation decisions a moral reference point, extending not only beyond oneself but specifically to the group of which everyone is a part. They provide a way to talk about a system to which *I* belong, and can in principle affirm, even when it endorses treatment practices different from those that meet my own personal needs.

For example, suppose I learn that I will die for lack of a new liver because outcome studies indicate that patients with my physiologic frailties are poor risks for this very expensive therapy, and I also find out that the calculations show that this money is best spent on nutritional programs for pregnant teenagers. I at least have a moral reference point that relates me and my needs to others and their needs, and to the priorities of a social order. It is one of the pernicious aspects of the current U.S. system that needs, even easily treatable ones, are isolated burdens, and their ranking for treatment or non-treatment cannot be referenced to any perceptible social good. It is precisely this tangible moral reference for solidarity that principles of utility can provide.

At the same time, the personal aspects of health care needs cannot be collapsed into the requirements of utility. A health care system cannot adopt wholesale the population-based aims of public health. It must attend also to the need for private, therapeutic relationships without regard for overall efficiency. Personal demands for marginal or useless care can and have subverted aims of fair distribution by monopolizing services needed by others. However, a system that failed to recognize persons as individuals and responded only to categories of diseases in terms of their malleability would not be worth the resources required to sustain it. Any feasible health care system must strike a balance between impartial fairness in the service of the public good and personal recognition in the service of private goods. Yet as I will argue in subsequent chapters, public and private goods in health care are closely related.

Libertarian theories of justice would seem to be the most difficult to reconcile with the goals I propose, but they too should have a place in our thinking about health care. Libertarian views remind us that although security and solidarity are fundamental goals of a system, they are not its only values. These goals may, as I argue, override other concerns, but they do not obliterate them. Aiming for security and solidarity does tax liberty; it will likely restrict the training and practice opportunities of future physicians and the conditions for buying and selling health insurance, to cite just two examples. Keeping liberty interests in mind as we devise a better health care system should minimize the burden placed on individuals. It may also help to counter utopian aspirations of those who are too enamored of the benefits of a right to health care. Because it is innately suspicious of social entitlements, libertarianism should lead us to question the benefits of conceiving health care as a right and keep the positive content of any such right within clear limits. Libertarian theories are an important force for parsimony in the system.

The discussion of justice continues in Chapters 3 and 4, but in a different way. In this chapter I have been concerned about theories of justice as methodological tools, concepts to test experiences and intuitions, to sharpen the inquiry into purpose and goals. In the following chapters I am concerned to explore the *motives* for justice, that is, those forces which will impel us to embrace the goals I have defined, and the view of persons and society that undergird them.

CHAPTER THREE

Self-Interest and Security:

A Humean Contract for Health Care

It is one thing to assert that the goals of security and solidarity should be the defining purpose of health care and the aims of a just system. It is another thing to make convincing arguments. Why should anyone, and especially the well-insured, embrace these goals? Answering this question is the task to which I now turn.

This chapter is devoted to developing the insights of David Hume and applying them to the issue of health care. Hume argued that just institutions develop from self-interest. I will argue that self-interest must be recognized as a key element in the effort to institute a system of universal care, and that it is crucial for linking the goals of security and solidarity. Chapter 4 continues this line of argument by discrediting atomistic views of the self. These views, by denying the importance of human affinities and social relationships, distort the ways in which we define self-interest. Together these two chapters show that security and solidarity are not only desirable but attainable.

A chapter that emphasizes self-interest can perhaps be forgiven for beginning on a personal note. I assume my experience is typical and therefore can serve as a familiar example of current problems with health insurance.

Over the past six years my health insurance premiums have risen at an average rate of more than 20 percent annually, while my policy has diminished appreciably in value. The co-insurance (that part of my hospital and physician bills I pay myself) has increased from 10 percent to 20 percent, and the maximum co-insurance has been increased. The deductible (the part I pay before my insurance coverage begins) has gone from $100 to $250 per year per person. I am told my coverage is good and I should be grateful. I am also warned that health insurance costs for state employees and university faculty in North Carolina will increase by $150–170 million next year, which means that the legislature will likely be forced to choose (again) between granting pay increases and retaining the current level of health care benefits. Even if the level of benefits is retained, the co-payments and deductibles will likely increase again.

My children, young adults now and launching their own lives, have repeatedly passed in and out of eligibility for coverage under my policy for the past several years, depending upon their age, student status, and other factors. This has necessitated the purchase of policies with high premiums and low benefits to insure their care, and to protect me from the burden of potentially crushing expenses should they need extensive amounts of care. Such policies typically do not cover routine outpatient services, and most require a twelve-month period of exemption for "pre-existing conditions," a term which I fear would be defined in ways advantageous to insurers rather than to me.

This escalation in costs for diminished value in health insurance is not, however, the most distressing aspect of the current scene. The real problem is the larger pattern and what it portends. While my health insurance costs have been rising at an annual rate averaging more than 20 percent, the general inflationary rate has been roughly 4 percent, and my salary has risen at an even more modest rate. At the current rate of growth my insurance premiums will exceed $1,200 per month before the turn of the century.

This is not a litany of complaint, for I do feel fortunate, especially in comparison with friends who have been laid off in "downsizing" business maneuvers and have lost their health insurance altogether, or in comparison with those who have never had insurance. Rather, this is testimony to a growing sense of vulnerability among many Americans right now, including those of us with "good jobs." It is the feeling of being personally at risk, which is different from a more general awareness of the problems plaguing the U.S. health care system. A personal sense of risk changes the stakes, and should change the way we (the insured) reason about justice in health care and what will motivate us toward health care reform.

This chapter seeks to articulate one powerful, self-interested reason for supporting universal health care. It does not seek to be exhaustive, or exclusive. The self-interested arguments for universal care are many, and the reasons for embracing an inclusive system extend beyond self-interested motives. Nevertheless, reasoning from self-interest seems especially important. If universal health care can be shown to be in everyone's, or almost everyone's, concrete and readily perceived self-interest, appeals to our sense of altruism will not have to bear the entire burden of moving us toward a more just system.

Instability and Insecurity

Instability is not always found on the list of problems that currently plague health care, but it belongs near the top. Few people can be confident that their access to affordable care is invulnerable to sudden change. Insurance costs now preempt wage increases. Employers are shifting health costs to workers, greatly increasing the costs of premiums as well as the level of co-insurance and deductibles. Many workers fear changing jobs because of the risk of losing their insurance altogether, a phenomenon commonly referred to as "job lock." Insurers routinely devise new ways to avoid the sick. Hospitals now employ experts to teach them to "game" the reimbursement systems to make a profit and to avoid unprofitable patients. These maneuvers on the part of insurers and hospitals may seem appalling, but they should be expected: in today's system of economic competition, avoidance of the uninsured patient or the low-reimbursement case is the price of success. But the point here is not the usual moralizing one about social Darwinism in health care; the issue is the lack of stability in the current system. Dan Beauchamp and Henry Aaron, among others, have argued that the stability issue is central, but it has not been a prominent ingredient in discussions of health care reform.[1] Clearly it should be.

Most people with health insurance have little assurance that they will not at some point join the 37 million other Americans who are uninsured. Moreover, the figure of 37 million is misleading; it is misleading as an overestimate of unmet needs, because many of these persons are healthy young adults, and misleading as an underestimate of those lacking true security, because if the underinsured are included among those who are vulnerable the number is closer to 70 million persons.[2] The underinsured are those for whom a major illness with an extensive hospital stay would be economically ruinous.

Those who have adequate health insurance but who work for self-insured employers have another kind of risk. The Employee Retirement and Income Security Act of 1974 (ERISA) gives self-insured businesses an exemption from state health insurance regulations. Such businesses have great discretionary power in deciding what to cover, and they may reduce insurance coverage after the onset of an illness. This makes self-insurance attractive to an employer seeking to reduce costs but leaves employees vulnerable. Reductions in the maximum insurance coverage from $1 million to $10,000 for persons diagnosed with HIV infection have been reported, and the legality of these reductions has been confirmed by the courts. In 1985, 58 percent of all employers were self-insured, and this percentage is likely even higher now.[3] Because it is the larger employers that self-insure, the percentage of employees who are covered by self-insured plans is much higher than 58 percent. Thus, the ERISA exemptions have made people usually considered well-insured much more vulnerable than is commonly recognized.

Moreover, in the future the disadvantages for individuals in a risk-based insurance system will be compounded by an increase in genetic testing. Genetic information is now routinely used by insurers, but the amount of useful information that can be obtained from genetic screening is small. Thomas H. Murray suggests that research in human genetics, such as the Human Genome Project, "is likely to increase dramatically our ability to predict whether individuals are at risk for particular diseases."[4] Murray argues that actuarial fairness, what he terms a "Lloyds of London" model, is not a good model for fairness in health insurance since it divides the world into the well and the sick (or potentially sick) and undermines the social purpose of providing health insurance. Yet fair or not, the actuarial model is increasingly the model used in decisions about access to and cost of health insurance.

Health insurance no longer means assured access to services, or payment for services rendered. Instability, and the insecurity it generates, is a central aspect of our predicament, and it must be recognized as such by the well-insured, self-interested person, whom I am addressing here.

A Humean Contract

Perceived insecurity as the motive force for justice was given definitive modern expression by David Hume. In both *A Treatise of Human Nature* and in the second *Enquiry,* Hume maintained that just institutions arise in human societies because we come to understand that our own property will not be secure unless we respect the property of others. Hume believed that each of us is naturally partial to ourselves and to our family and friends, and this partiality in our affections influences not only our behavior but also our natural sense of right and wrong. Thus anyone who gave preference to a stranger over his family or friends would be seen as lacking in virtue. Yet while this partiality in our sympathy is proper, it would, if taken alone, leave us unfit for life in society. The remedy for "unequal affection," or partiality, as Hume saw it, is not the counterbalancing of self-interest by another sentiment, like benevolence, but adherence to learned responses based on an assessment of where our true interest lies.[5]

It is in this sense that Hume referred to justice as an "artificial" virtue. "Artificial" does not mean that justice is an arbitrary or capricious value, just that it is an invention of society rather than an instinctive part of human nature. The advantages of justice come to us through "judgment and understanding." Hume put it with characteristic directness in the *Treatise:* "I observe, that it will be for my interest to leave another in the possession of his goods, *provided* he will act in the same manner with regard to me. He is sensible of a like interest in the regulation of his conduct. When this common sense of interest is mutually express'd, and is known to both, it produces a suitable resolution and behavior."[6] The second *Enquiry* echoes this formulation: "We are naturally partial to ourselves, and to our friends; but are capable of learning the advantage resulting from a more equitable conduct."[7]

Hume did not see justice as in any way an outgrowth of benevolence. Many of Hume's contemporaries, influenced by theological notions of altruism or charity, conceived of the moral life as a struggle between self-interest and benevolence. They believed only the ascendancy of benevolence would assure just institutions. Hume's view of human nature was less aspirational and more practical. "Tis certain," he confidently asserted, "that no affection of the human mind has both a sufficient force, and a proper direction to counter-balance the love of gain, and render men fit members of society, by making them abstain from the possessions of others." Benevolence is present in human nature, as Hume saw it, but is not powerful. What controls self-interest is greater self-interest. What counteracts the exercise of immediate self-interest is the recognition that long-range self-interest requires justice: "the passion [self-love] is much better satisfy'd by its restraint, than by its liberty."[8]

Given this formulation of how we arrive at justice, Hume believed that it makes little difference whether we think of self-interest as a vice or a virtue, since its workings, for the person of understanding, will lead to the same result. The powerful sense we all have that justice is virtuous springs not from our natural affections, he thought, since just acts often require that we sometimes go against our own natural partiality. Rather, the desire for justice as a moral ideal results from our sympathy with others, which enables us to identify, and identify with, a public good. Thus, although we arrive at justice through a calculation of self-interest, the hold that justice has on us is magnified because of our social passions and our tendencies to seek affiliations with others. Here our self-love and our less powerful fellow-feeling, or sympathy with others, coincide. The virtuous appearance of justice is, then, taken up and magnified in the discourse of parents, teachers, clergy, and politicians. The result is a system of customs (and, later, rules) of justice that make for a stable society in which individuals are secure in their property.

The arguments Hume made for possessions in the mid-eighteenth century also apply to health care in the late twentieth century. To paraphrase Hume, "I observe that it will be in my interest to support others in their access to health services, provided they will act in a similar manner with regard to me." Universal access is, then, perceived as the way to secure continued access to my own care. Solidarity with others in developing and supporting a system of universal care is the path to security. I cannot expect to gain or retain access to health care unless others have the same opportunity; put more practically, I cannot expect to bend the health system to my will to the detriment of others and anticipate that they will refrain from using resources that I may also need. What is at issue is the security of my person, which can only be assured if my access (now linked to everyone's) to needed care can be assured.

It could be objected here that the "Humean" arrangement is one that the well-insured will want to make only with each other. Those who are uninsured cannot share this motivation to protect their secure access to care, for they have none. But this way of thinking assumes that "the well-insured" and "the medically indigent" are stable categories. As we have seen, in the current climate the well-insured can and do quickly become medically indigent. The precariousness of insurability means that both insured and uninsured already belong together in the same risk pool. The extraordinary cost of health care means that what is at stake is not just the security of access to health care but the security of one's person, and of one's property more generally. The threat of medical insecurity is not just the threat of being denied care but the threat of being impoverished by the help one does receive. This is the plight of the underinsured. The plight of the chronically or seriously ill is that they will become uninsurable.

These threats endanger all of us. Health care is so intertwined with our general well-being, both physically and materially, that health insurance cannot be separated out as an incidental possession. So the implication of Humean thinking for the late twentieth century is that everyone must be assured access to health care if I am to retain mine. The "common sense of interest ... mutually express'd" must include the medically indigent because, in practical terms of both property and person, the well-insured and the indigent are now equally vulnerable.

A Humean social contract for health care based on a common need for security should be distinguished from a Hobbesian contract based on fear. While both Hume and Hobbes emphasized insecurity, there are important differences between them. Fear plays a central, almost exhaustive, role in Hobbes's philosophy. Hume held a more complex view. He saw human nature as both self-interested and altruistic, and as possessing instinctive social affinities, which help establish and sustain just institutions. The self-interest of Hume's ethics is a prudent self-regard, only one of a variety of passions and motives. The self-interest of Hobbes is an individualized and monolithic egoism. There is no doubt that the effect of our current health policies on many citizens is to make life, as in Hobbes's words, "solitary, poor, nasty, brutish and short."[9] As cost continues to escalate and access continues to diminish, insecurity turns to fear and Hobbes's description becomes more accurate. Yet Hume is a better spokesman for the sort of contract we now need in health care, because he accounts more completely for the complexity of human motives and experiences.

Other problems beyond the cost and access bode ill for our common health security. For example, in New York, Atlanta, Miami, and other areas of the country there is a resurgence of tuberculosis, indeed, drug-resistant strains of TB.[10] For over thirty years little attention had been paid to this disease because it was a problem only for the poor. TB may have persisted among our impoverished citizens because of a lack of medical attention and the improper or incomplete use of antibiotics, or perhaps because of poor nutrition and poor health status generally; the exact causes are irrelevant to my point. Finally, it was not thought to be important to eradicate tuberculosis, or in many cases even to detect its presence. It was acceptable for the poor to harbor TB; the rest of us were safe. Now we are all reaping the harvest of our neglect. Hospitals are ill-equipped to keep TB patients in the "negative pressure" isolation rooms that prevent infection of other patients and health care workers. Instead of the few millions of dollars it would have required to detect and eradicate the residues of TB in the poor a few years ago, it now will take hundreds of millions of dollars to protect the well and discover the new antibiotics required to treat the growing number of sick. The new TB epidemic, superimposed over the AIDS epidemic, is just one indication that, at least in health care, we cannot isolate our self-interest and make trade-offs against the needs of others. The needs of others are not distant objects of my philanthropy but part of my own security.

Security is of two sorts: economic and psychological. Economic security means that we have budgetary limits that make costs predictable and services sustainable over time. Psychological security means that we believe that the system is fair, that it is independent of political fortune, and that it will, consequently, remain in place over our lifetime. In psychological terms, security is represented by confidence in the system. We have none of this at present.

The ultimate aim is to forge a loyalty to a pattern of distribution of health services that is economically viable and widely affirmed as just. The alternative for most of us is a Humean insecurity (or Hobbesian angst) over whether I will become number 37-million-and-one. We cannot escape the stability question in health care in either its economic or psychological forms. It ultimately redounds to the question of whether we will have a safe and stable social order.

It is always possible that the response to insecurity will not be one of enlightened self-interest but a more primitive and tribal reaction. The immediate reaction to our insecurity may lead us not to work toward solidarity but to huddle together more tightly with our peer group, to work the health care system harder in our favor, and to exclude others more severely. This will lead to a quicker demise of the current arrangements, for it will make differences between the haves and have-nots progressively more obvious and brutal while accentuating the vulnerability of the system as a whole.

Self-Interest in Hume and Rawls

Many readers will recognize here a position similar to that developed by John Rawls in *A Theory of Justice*.[11] Rawls presents what is arguably the most influential contractarian approach to justice in this century, and in his approach self-interest plays an important role. Yet there is at least one crucial difference between a Rawlsian contract and the (Humean) scenario for a health care system as I have constructed it. While Rawls begins with contractors who are choosing from behind a veil of ignorance, without knowing their real situation, we are all too aware of our vulnerability.

Rawls's work has been frequently criticized for situating his original contractors behind a veil of ignorance.[12] Such contractors, it is argued, are too thinly drawn. Characterized only by prudence and rationality, they present moral agency asocially, ahistorically, and incompletely. Others have argued in reply that Rawls never intended the original contractors to represent moral agency, and that the asocial and ahistorical character of the contractors is a strategic advantage. As Charles Dougherty says, the point of a hypothetical contract, such as Rawls devises, is to separate our better selves from the biases associated with knowledge of our present circumstances. "The device of a veil of ignorance is meant to shut out the knowledge that makes bias and self-serving choices possible and inevitable."[13]

I do not wish to argue for or against Rawls, or hypothetical contract theory, but only to indicate how a Humean contract can enlarge and deepen our thinking. In doing so, I do not assume that Hume's views are ultimately the correct ones. Nor do I assume that anyone who adopts his perspective is committed to a utilitarian foundation for universal health care. These positions would require larger and more complex arguments. My goal is simply to show that whatever philosophical theory we may espouse, or even if we espouse no particular theory at all, a Humean perspective may be helpful in moving us toward universal care.

The appeal of Hume is that he speaks to persons as they commonly are, with rudimentary social instincts, a limited altruism, and a prudential self-regard. As a skeptic and an empiricist, Hume was unimpressed by arguments that would let us start over and reformulate the grounds of justice from ideal beginnings, or from only a few select human characteristics. He believed we know only too clearly who and where we are. He saw the particulars of our self-interest as constituting who we are, shaping how we will choose and how we will want to choose. In health care this means that those who are currently well-insured will not forget that fact when they think of health care reform. The idea that the well-insured will altruistically give up some of their medical care, or pay more for it, to benefit others is unrealistic. It is inconsistent with observed, human experiences, or as James Todd of the American Medical Association put it, "no one wants to pay higher taxes to help someone else."[14]

A Humean approach to health care reform will not depend too heavily either on benevolence or on a notion of fairness that asks us to set aside our concrete circumstances and adopt a disinterested point of view. Justice speaks to self-interest, Hume said, and grows out of it, though it develops into something larger and more virtuous. Initially, a Humean approach will emphasize to the well-insured how vulnerable they are, and how their vulnerability is linked with that of others, not what ideals should be espoused to assist the impoverished. In other words, a Humean approach seeks to arrive at universal care through reflection on common experience, not on the ideal conditions of choice.

Hume also emphasized the naturalness of social life and built this instinctual sociality into civic as well as personal morality. Society is made up not of discrete individuals but of families and kinship units, as well as affiliations of work and pleasure. Hume had no objection to state-of-nature social contract arguments, so long as they were recognized as "mere philosophical fiction."[15] The actual first state of human life, Hume asserted, was familial. "Man, born in a family, is compelled to maintain society, from necessity, from natural inclination, and from habit."[16] Because sociality is natural, social cohesiveness does not depend entirely on acts of will or deliberate choice but on "necessity," "inclination," and "habit." The principles of justice, then, need not rest only on hypothetical assent; judgments about turning human appetites and proclivities toward social purposes support the same principles. Hume's view has the merit of making the principles of social organization, including organized provision for health services, more directly related to concrete experience. Justice—though "artificial" in the Humean sense that it does not result from a specific instinct—is natural in the sense that it is "as immutable as human nature," or an outgrowth of our native sociality.[17] Justice originates not in benevolent tendencies but in self-consciousness about our own self-interest in an inextricably social world.

Benevolence and Justice: The Wall and the Vault

Benevolence, Hume says, is like a wall, "built by many hands, which still rises by each stone that is heaped upon it." Justice, by contrast, is like a vault, "where each individual stone would, of itself, fall to the ground" were it not for "the mutual assistance and combination of its corresponding parts."[18]

Benevolence and justice are different virtues, with different requirements and different results. Each act of benevolence is self-contained, its motivation immediate and self-evident, its result apparent. The wall of benevolence, constructed of the stones of separate acts, may be short, but the size of the wall can always be increased by increment because the results are cumulative. No one good act depends upon any other. Justice, by contrast, depends upon a social self-consciousness, a sense of interdependence. Benevolence is social in the sense that it involves relationships with others, but it does not require a recognition of interdependence. Justice cannot exist without a mutually held sense of what is good based ultimately on what is fair to all. As Hume says, justice must be self-conscious because just actions are sometimes contrary to our immediate self-interest, and some even run counter to the immediate interests of others. Justice, which is of great consequence for our long-term interests, requires that we acknowledge our interdependence and perhaps sacrifice some short-term benefits. Hence, justice is social in a more profound way than benevolence. Unlike the wall of benevolence, with its discrete and separable units, a just institution, like a vault, stands or falls as a whole.

Hume's imagery serves as another illustration of why no just health care system will ever result from benevolence alone. Justice in health care will no more result from the cumulative sum of independent benevolent acts than a vault can be created by piling stones one upon the other. One flaw of our past thinking about health care is the idea that we would have a fair system where all are cared for if only doctors, hospitals, and insurers were somehow more benevolent. Clearly this is not the case.

While benevolent actions no doubt contribute to the common good, they wax and wane with our sense of affluence and our feelings of generosity toward others. Justice is a product of enlightened self-interest and socially recognized cooperation for long-term benefit, not selfless regard for the good of others. A system based solely on benevolence is unstable not only because of fluctuation in the good will of the powerful, but also because no reciprocal arrangements exist to cement the separate acts into a social structure. Like a vault, a health care system is made stable by inclusiveness.

The American experience demonstrates Hume's point. Benevolence is too limited a force in the moral psyche to move us, by itself, to a just system of universal care. Yet even if it were sufficient, there may be good reason to avoid it as the chief impetus for health care reform. Benevolent actions reflect the virtue and generosity of the doers but require little of the recipients, except to display their neediness and offer gratitude. But the receivers of benevolently given goods may also feel resentment because the care received is understood by both giver and receiver to be a gift—a gift it is impossible to repay—and resentment compounds material advantage of the donor with the presumption of a moral superiority.[19] Largesse is an exchange between unequals. In short, the absence of reciprocity in a system driven solely by benevolence runs the risk of further damaging the self-esteem of the recipients and threatens to breed resentment. A system of universal care based on appeals to the self-interest of the insured will be more sound, morally and psychologically, and thereby more durable.

Objections

Some may object that appeals to self-interest are frequently convincing but that they have nothing to do with ethics. Ethics, they might say, is designed to give us reasons for overriding our self-interest. Being a moral person is, precisely, forgoing our self-interest and acting altruistically.

This is a popular but faulty view. Its popularity likely stems from (misreadings of) religious teachings that urge total selflessness and love for one's neighbors. It is faulty because it denies any value to having concern for one's self. Such a truncated view of ethics is unsound because impractical. While selfless love of one's neighbor is admirable, it is difficult to find anyone who can consistently practice it. Moreover, as Jane Mansbridge puts it, "normative systems that make self-interest morally unacceptable also make it hard, if not impossible, to recognize and handle those self-interested impulses that continue to exist."[20] Selfless motivation should be affirmed but not assumed to present a complete picture of human capacities, and clearly not one on which to build policy. For Hume a proportionate self-interest is not morally neutral; it is a positive virtue, a thing to be praised and emulated. Self-interest—at least in Hume's sense—does not mean a calculating egoism but a prudent self-regard. The task of ethics is not to suppress or deny self-interest but to enlighten our conception of it through reason and demonstrate its connection with social virtues. The great enemy of just institutions is not self-interest but an ignorant or egoistical self-interest—one not sufficiently grounded in social reciprocity.

Some will be disappointed that this analysis does not have a more central place for community; no doubt some believe that any analysis of health care problems must presuppose and begin with a communal perspective. It is true that one cannot begin with an atomistic notion of persons and arrive at a viable sense of community, as I will argue in the next chapter. Still, it takes too much for granted to use the word *community* as an accurate description of our current situation in health care. In fact we are currently separated by many factors: genetic and environmental conditions, age-specific and disease-specific programs for the delivery of care, as well as health insurance status. Frequently the differences in access and entitlements reflect differences in income and race. It is true, to be sure, that these factors, generally seen as forces of separation, might also be seen as a means of binding us to others. Genetic conditions, for example, link us to family members; environmental pollutants make foul the air and water for all of us; and even age is a connecting factor, since most of us will pass through the same life stages. My point is not that we have no basis for community consciousness but that in health policy the forces linking us together are currently far less powerful than the forces keeping us apart. In the end, a communitarian perspective is essential, but we cannot begin with it as an assumption.

Many Americans seem to have only enough sense of community to sustain a working relationship with those nearest to them; we function largely in work-related, religious, residential, or recreational enclaves. The sense of a broader identity, such as belonging to a political entity and sharing the benefits and burdens of citizenship, is undoubtedly present, but has not been employed to date to forge health policies that are equitable and sustainable. Robert Reich observes that the idea of community has a special attraction for Americans, but that it is so narrowly defined that "generosity and solidarity end at the borders of our common property values."[21] This observation seems to me unarguable, and is the reason that this chapter assumes the necessity to speak first to self-interest and not beg the issues by relying primarily or completely on a broad, benevolent, communitarian orientation as a basis for action. Analyses of the health care problem that are built on a strong and taken-for-granted sense of community make the task too easy, and they too frequently begin and end with hortatory remarks about the virtues of belonging. The questions of what we belong to in health care, and what would be worth belonging to, are the central questions—they cannot be begged. Rather than assuming community as the foundational element in our arguments, we should look to a universal health care system to help develop a greater sense of community.

All realistic alternatives for reform will at least not be inconsistent with self-interest. In health care, personal self-interest eventually involves the good of others. Our needs and rewards in life more generally are not ours alone, except perhaps for winning the lottery or the Nobel Prize. For a great many of life's goods, there is an inextricable link between my well-being and that of others. This is especially true in health care. The appeal of communitarian altruism is important in health care reform, but it is not sufficient, and it is not a good point of origin. Self-interest, far from being an inhospitable ground for universal care, is a necessary basis for it.

Some might object that relying on self-interest will make it difficult to select the package of services that would be available to all. For example, suppose that I know that no one in my family, or my spouse's family, has a history of schizophrenia. Because this disease has a genetic component, I can be fairly certain that no one in my family is likely to develop schizophrenia. Treating schizophrenia is expensive, involving not only medical but social support that may be required for decades. Choosing from self-interest, therefore, I will not want to have this disease included in the benefits package available in a universal health care system. The same argument could be made for many diseases that have a strong genetic component. For example, many homeless persons are mentally ill. One could argue, perhaps, that because these persons live in the streets, subway stations, bus terminals, and other public places they jeopardize my security in ways other than my access to health care, so it is therefore in my self-interest for the chronically mentally ill to be cared for. But this is a dubious argument, given the high cost of medical treatment in comparison with public health or safety measures. At this point it might be thought that self-interest has run its course and that we must resort to our sense of benevolence to argue for adequate care for everyone.

I would agree that self-interest is not the only virtue in a well-formed ethic; moreover, I would agree that benevolence is an essential ingredient for any workable social program. But I resist the idea that caring for the poor and disenfranchised hinges primarily or entirely on benevolence because the well-insured have nothing (or, as we are prone to say, nothing "personally") at risk in the current system.

The problem in this way of thinking lies in the effort to single out one disease, or one pattern of illness episodes, as an example while leaving all other health problems unexamined. What can be said about genetic predisposition and schizophrenia can also be said about occupational predispositions and illnesses, or race and illnesses, and so on. For example, secretarial work requiring long hours of typing (such as preparing the various drafts of this manuscript) predisposes persons to carpel tunnel syndrome. Medicine and dentistry, for reasons that are unclear, are associated with high rates of depression, drug addiction, and suicide. Would it be in my self-interest as a university professor to exclude these illnesses from the universal package because I am not at high risk for them? Should I exclude sickle-cell disease because I am not African-American? If so, I must worry that secretaries, doctors and dentists, or African-Americans will discover a correlation between my work, race, life-style, or genetic makeup that will make me a health care undesirable. This mutual suspicion would obviously undermine the sense of security we want from a universal system. So, to interpret Hume at the level of specifying a benefits package, the "common sense of interest . . . mutually express'd" is that no one will seek to exclude others on the basis of health care needs that arise because of such differences. It is in my interest to support benefits for others that I am unlikely to use, for only by so doing can I expect them to support programs that I might need but they would not. And we should not forget that predictions of what anyone is likely to need are notoriously unreliable. Finally, the picking and choosing of benefits as suggested above would simply replicate the sense of insecurity we feel in the face of experience-based indemnity health insurance.

This problem of partial inclusion relates to persons as well as diseases. For example, it is possible that the current system could be reformed in such a way to include most people but not everyone. This large majority might feel secure enough that their self-interest would not be threatened by the suffering of those left out. If the excluded group were thought to be powerless, and if one's inclusion were a matter of entitlement, then keeping the doors of access shut might seem more prudent than opening them to the excluded few. Moreover, rationalizations for continuing to exclude those on the outside seem endless. The "others" might be characterized as having brought illness upon themselves, as not really desiring care, as not knowing how to use health services, as having abused their access to resources, and so on. One need only look at the rationales for the inequitable arrangements we now have to see the possibilities. Our power to excuse ourselves from what we take to be optional, benevolent actions is enormous.

Yet partial inclusion of persons would fail for much the same reason that partial inclusion of diseases would fail. Namely, the sense of security it would give is a false one, as can be illustrated by the difficulties any system of health care faces. Not only is there the risk of falling out of the included into the excluded category, which should make any reflective person pause. There are also the inevitable adjustments that must be made because health care services continue to be expensive relative to other goods and services. It would be naive to think that any entitlement to health benefits would not need future adjustments. If the system already contained a precedent for exclusion, however small, it is easy to see how coverage for, say, 95 percent of the population could turn into coverage for 85 percent in difficult times. In the matter of health services, security is an all-or-nothing affair. A health care system is either universal or it is not. If it is not, the door is always open to the possibility of dealing with cost overruns by taking people out of the system. This is precisely the most prevalent method for dealing with cost overruns in the Medicaid program to date, as each state, mandated to provide specific services to those who are eligible, adjusts its eligibility requirements to meet its budget.

Finally, it could be objected that the difficulty of assuring mutual support is a major problem for a system based on self-interest. The Humean formulation states that it is in my self-interest to support others in their access to health care *provided* they will act in a similar manner with regard to me. How do I know that this provision will be fulfilled? What assurance do I have that at least sufficient numbers will reciprocate my support for them? If persons were to act as social atoms, each striving to make separate contracts with all the others, this would indeed be a problem. Yet one of the purposes of government is to carry out the public will in matters that individuals, acting separately, cannot organize or execute for themselves. I take it to be one of the functions of government to assure universal participation in a health care system. This requires not only regulative authority, but moral authority. The President—among others—must lead, teach, and exhort participation on civic grounds as well as health grounds. I will have more to say about the civic meaning of universal care at a later point. For now, I simply note that the assurance of participation and setting of standards is one role government can and must play in establishing a system of universal care.

In summary, Hume's conception of justice has several things to recommend it in our efforts to reform the health care system in the direction of universal care.

First, it engages us concretely rather than hypothetically, and its appeal is therefore more direct and immediate. It appeals to what we know about ourselves, rather than asking us to suspend this self-knowledge as morally arbitrary. It may present problems of bias, as Rawls and others have indicated, but given the continuing deterioration of health benefits for the insured, this is less a problem now than it was a few years ago, and is steadily diminishing in force.

Second, by emphasizing self-interest, Hume bypasses problems of insufficient benevolence, or limited altruism. The picture of moral life he presents is less flattering but more realistic than many of the alternative views of the human condition.

Third, Hume's views are best seen not as a replacement for hypothetical contracts for justice made by choice, but as a supplement to them. One of Hume's signal contributions to ethics lies in his moral psychology and the practicality of his portrait of moral agency. His contribution to the debate about health care reform is his perceptiveness about the motives for justice. If we can set aside hankerings for a canonical and all-embracing theory, there is no reason we cannot combine this Humean empiricism with a Rawlsian, or other, approach. As I argued earlier, each major theory of justice may well benefit the debate. The moral foundations for universal health care are multiple, but we would do well to give Humean self-interest a primary place in our arguments.

CHAPTER FOUR

Affinity and Solidarity:

Getting from I to We

In the previous chapter I rejected the strategy of making assumptions about community the basis of reform and argued for universal care on grounds of self-interest. Community consciousness is an important force, indeed, a necessary element in any feasible health care system, but to make it a first premise begs too many questions. A cooperative and inclusive sense of community is a goal of health policy, not its foundation. The aim is solidarity—not the organic relatedness of a Gemeinschaft but the more rational reciprocity of a Gesellschaft. Rational, cooperative interactions are not devoid of benevolence and, in health care especially, they can be fertile ground in which benevolent attitudes may grow and flourish. Yet a sense of community is not contingent upon benevolence as a foundation. This is the lesson of Hume for health care.

Still, developing even this more modest sense of solidarity will not be simple, for standing in the way are traditions of social and moral atomism. As Charles Taylor puts it, "atomist views always seem nearer to common sense, more immediately available," and unless we make a special effort, "we tend to fall back into an atomist/instrumentalist way of seeing."[1] My task in this chapter is to make that special effort, to examine atomism critically and indicate an alternative. As I will show, it is impossible to move from atomistic beginnings to a social view of persons; to adopt atomism is to foreclose on solidarity from the start. Given my emphasis on self-interest, it is especially important to show that the self who discerns his or her interest is not an atomistic self. My intention is not to refute atomism thoroughly but to display its weaknesses and put a more realistic conception of self and society on exhibit, namely, one that accounts for the natural affinities and sympathies of human association. Here again the argument will rely on a reading of Hume, with the addition of advances made upon Hume's moral philosophy by Adam Smith.

Atomism: Beginning with *I*

Amitai Etzioni claims that "the celebration of individualism has been carried too far, beyond the challenge of authoritarian and totalitarian doctrines, to undercutting the legitimation of the community and of the public realm."[2]

His response is not a return to community in a simplistic sense, but to what he terms, following Martin Buber, "I and We," or the "Open Community." Etzioni sees traditional conservative conceptions of the community as closed and inimical to individual rights, and traditional liberal conceptions as noncommunal, and sometimes anticommunal. The Open Community is one in which communal and individual forces both have standing and in which the tension between them is valued as a healthy dynamic, not viewed as a problem to be solved. The moral force of both the individual and the community is anchored in its response to its opposite. Traditional conservative and liberal positions, the "closed community" and "no community" options, collapse the tension and force this dynamic into a rigid (and thereby unstable) resolution.

It is something very close to Etzioni's model that I want to endorse here. Yet, much of our moral and social language steers away from this sort of dynamic synthesis of the multiple sides of our moral selves in favor of more simplistic formulations of both the problem and its possible solutions. The predominant American political ethic is liberal, or "no community," in orientation: we put a heavy emphasis on individual rights and liberties, and we tend to be suspicious that all forms of community are authoritarian and repressive.

Alternatives to atomism of great intellectual force could be cited here, and the issues could be engaged in a deliberative fashion. Yet the reason atomism has had such a powerful, almost captivating influence in the West may have less to do with its intellectual persuasiveness and more to do with the emotional appeal of its portrait of the self. My argument here follows a line of thinking suggested by Charles Taylor.[3] The staying power of atomism, he argues, has to do with the seductive way it depicts the individual. The atomistic view emphasizes an individual's freedom, dignity, and power; in short, it portrays persons as moral sovereigns who are free to choose social relationships, or community affiliation, and whose lives remain essentially unchanged by such choices.

The portrait could be described roughly as follows: In the beginning (or "in the state of nature," or "behind the veil of ignorance," or "in the Garden") were individuals, and these discrete units were essentially complete unto themselves and self-sufficient with regard to their needs and aims. For reasons of convenience and mutual gain, these individuals decided to form social compacts. Included in these compacts were moral requirements indicating how each individual would relinquish some independence in exchange for the benefits of collective activity. Yet these social compacts were optional and provisional, and they in no way changed the essential and antecedent freedom, dignity, or power of each individual over him/herself. Each individual remained free to disengage from any particular social compact, or from all social compacts whatever, when the balance of self-interest versus the sacrifice of restrictions was not to the individual's advantage.

This formulation, frequently in modified form, has dominated our thinking for at least three hundred years, and arguably longer. We could use the publication of Locke's *Second Treatise on Government* in 1690 as a convenient benchmark. This portrait is hardly ever painted in such bold colors, but I have presented it so blatantly to bring out, not its logical persuasiveness or its realism (of which there is little), but its emotional appeal. Whether presented as history or as hypothetical vignette, as fact or as argumentative stipulation, it carries the same appeal to our psyche. The message is one of grandeur, freedom, dignity, and power. It is a portrait of a sovereign. Individual existence is essential to human beings, social existence optional. Individuals constitute the moral unit of meaning worthy of study. Social relations, being derivative, are ethically uninteresting except as they form an occasion for, or the setting of, individual moral choice. Social relations, much less communal existence, are not constitutive of persons, or of the morally important aspects of persons. This view, of course, tilts the study of ethics in a certain way. But more important than the theoretical skewing of a discipline is the flattering picture of the self offered by the atomistic philosophy.

Moving to *We*

It should not be surprising that modern political philosophy should begin with atomism and move to a construction of society based on individual choice. Modern epistemology had already cut the path. Descartes put it definitively when he asserted that "I think, therefore I am."[4] The impact of this pronouncement for our view of knowledge has been enormous. Of equal importance is the form of the assertion for our moral self-understanding. Descartes did not say, from the solitariness of his Dutch oven, "We think, therefore we are,"—or, better, "We are, therefore I think." He said "I," not as Etzioni would have had it, "I and We," just "I"—a sovereign, essentially asocial self. Descartes said that in matters of knowledge the mind begins with itself and proceeds to the outside world through inference and construction. Modern political philosophy, following suit, begins with moral and social atomism and proceeds to the larger world through choice and construction.

In the best of all worlds we might hope for a reformulation something like, "We are, therefore I am able to think," to signal the roots of individual self-awareness in the soil of sociality. If we could acknowledge our debt to sociality we could then assert, "I think, therefore we are," to signal the crucial way that individuals must sustain communal activity.

I do not gainsay the importance of individual liberation, historically, from repressive collectivities or tyrannical political hierarchies. But I believe we can still maintain individual freedoms while embracing social affiliations. We need not sacrifice the dignity, power, and freedom we wish to ascribe to individuals; the solution is to situate them socially, as features of our social selves. Yet a good deal of current thinking portrays individual freedom and social relatedness as mutually exclusive, as if one must choose between them.

Atomistic predilections in the field of bioethics are most clearly indicated by preoccupation with the concept of autonomy. Concern for autonomy is proper and important—even vital—but it may sometimes diminish our appreciation for other values in health care, especially those of affiliation and fairness in allocation decisions. Respect for the autonomous health care choices of others, devoid of any sense of solidarity in how resources may fairly be used, is an unbalanced ethic. It extends autonomy (as a monolithic ideal) beyond the appropriate range of its application. For example, when elderly patients suffering multiple organ-system failure receive intensive services simply because it is thought to be their right to choose them, autonomy has become disproportionately valued. The countervailing needs of others for scarce resources are given no weight. Using autonomy as a moral "trump card" in situations for which it is ill-suited not only diminishes the importance of justice and other values, it ultimately warps the principle of autonomy as well. This is an understandable overextension of an ideal, given the traditions of atomism detailed above. An autonomy ethic of grandiose proportions fits all too neatly with the portrait of sovereignty inherited from Descartes and Locke.

In summary, if we begin with Cartesian certainty and Lockean self-sufficiency as the definitive picture of selfhood, we cannot get from I to We, for this I is a disengaged and essentially completed entity; it has no need to become part of a We. Cooperative relationships are always seen as a compromise of liberty. That such a portrait is false, or at best a distortion, and that we must begin with I *and* We, as Etzioni would have us say, is my point here. We cannot begin with a premise of asocial individualism and arrive at a viable social ethic. If there is to be a social ethic of any force, it must be discovered as a necessary complement to an individual ethic.

Sympathetic Exchanges: Locating I in We

As a contrast to the Cartesian-Lockean portrait of selves and society, consider the following scenario derived from Hume: The earliest experiences of humankind ("in the beginning") are social. They involve the succor and support of a family into which one is born and about which no choices are made. Of all members of the animal kingdom, humans are the least well equipped to care for themselves or function self-sufficiently. Affiliations and alliances are therefore a "necessity," a matter of survival throughout a person's life, but they also fulfill a natural inclination for affinity with others that is strengthened by habit and custom.

It follows that not only is the portrait of social and moral atomism endorsed by the Cartesian-Lockean paradigm false, in Hume's view, but it would be a kind of hell. Hume conceived a human being as "the creature of the universe who has the most ardent desire for society" and as "fitted for it by the most advantages." "We can form no wish," he said, "which has not a reference to society," and solitude and isolation would be "the greatest punishment we could suffer." Even if a person had power to make the sun rise and set or command the seas and rivers, Hume contended, "he will still be miserable, till you give him some one person at least, with whom he may share his happiness, and whose esteem and friendship he may enjoy."[5]

The name Hume often gave in his writings to this natural social affinity is *sympathy*, a term which was widely used in late-eighteenth-century Europe to designate what was thought to be an innate human capacity. Hume and Adam Smith were the most important exponents of sympathy, and rehearsing some of their thinking will assist us in locating the natural affinities on which a health care system can be built if we wish to achieve solidarity.

For Hume and Smith, sympathy designated not a feeling but a capacity for sharing feelings and experiences. Both claimed that this capacity is the foundation for (in the sense of the origin of) human moral experience. Hume called it the most remarkable quality of human nature and the chief source of moral distinctions.[6] He believed that other forms of animal life have this capacity as well, but humans have it to a much greater degree. It is understood as a mark of our nature as essentially social beings. Adam Smith held a similar view, but with important advances on Hume's thinking, which I will indicate shortly. Both philosophers conceived of sympathy as a basic human phenomenon— something that lies at the very roots of social affiliations, the deepest and impenetrable layer in the archeology of moral experience. Both Hume and Smith aspired to be the Isaac Newton of the human sciences. They thought of sympathy in the human world as like gravity in the natural world—a pervasive principle that accounts for the dynamics of social interaction.

Hume believed it was self-evident, what he called "the plainest experience," that people tend to reflect each other's feelings.[7] Being around those who are sad tends to make us feel sad; association with the joyous usually makes us so as well. Hume's descriptions of sympathy are typically of mundane experiences that are direct and unreflective. His metaphors for sympathy convey this same directness and immediacy. In one passage the minds of people are described as mirrors to each other, reflecting sentiments in reverberations, a sort of echo chamber of feeling.[8] In another passage persons are described "as strings equally wound," in which a motion in one is communicated to all the rest.[9]

The faculty of imagination plays a role, but a limited one. In a mechanical sense, imagination always plays a part in sympathy because it is the mechanism through which ideas become felt experiences. In a second way the imagination comes into play because we can and do sympathize with feelings not immediately presented to us but remote in time or place. For example, we can make ourselves feel sick from imagining what it would be like.[10] We feel anxiety and sorrow for those we think are about to be injured, and we can feel shame for someone who behaves foolishly, even if he is unaware that he is making a spectacle of himself.[11] Thus the imagination serves as a conduit for sympathetic responses but can also create such responses. Still, for Hume the imaginative capacity is tied to present stimuli. It can go beyond what is immediately offered to the senses, but when it does it tends to duplicate past experiences through association. Of course, this conception of imagination fits well into Hume's general empiricist doctrines and his philosophy of mind.

Smith gave to the workings of sympathy a broader and more complex dynamic. Whereas Humean sympathy was focused on pleasure or pain, Smith's notion of sympathy involved a sharing of any and all feelings.[12] Whereas Humean sympathy is typically direct and unmediated, Smith conceived it differently. To sympathize, on Smith's model, is to project ourselves imaginatively into another's *situation* and then to conceive what that person must be feeling. When a person is being tortured, for example, we do not feel what he feels but we "tremble and shudder at the thought of what he feels."[13]

Note two important differences here. First, in Smith's view we sympathize with *other people*, not with their feelings. Sympathy is about changing places, not just "mimicking" a feeling. Second, note the more sophisticated role given to imagination. Hume had a place for imagination also, but it took a lesser role, a role confined to the mental interior whereby ideas get lively enough to count as felt experiences. For Smith imagination is not an interior mental faculty but an external, social faculty whereby I can displace myself into another's shoes.

While some of Smith's examples suggest that sympathy can be automatic and unreflective, other examples indicate that sympathy often requires some real work.[14] This effort is necessary because sympathy is not what I would feel if I were in your place but what I imagine you must be feeling, given who you are, in your particular and unique circumstances. Thus, if I sympathize with you over the loss of your child, I do not sympathize by analogy, and ask myself, "If I had a child, how would I feel if I lost her?" Rather, my sympathy stretches out to you and your loss of this particular child, and the loss it is for you. It is this real extension to others that keeps sympathy from being just a sophisticated version of narcissism. Indeed, in a remarkable passage criticizing the egoistic philosophies of Hobbes and Mandeville, Smith offers the intriguing suggestion that those who reduce all ethical motives to self-love must have been tempted to do so because they recognized the importance of sympathy but misunderstood its workings.[15]

Effort is required in another way as well, as Smith recognizes in us a desire for mutual sympathy, which is not just consonance of feeling but a self-consciousness of this consonance. So while as observers we work to imagine what others feel, those being observed tend to modulate their feelings in appreciation of what an observer can imagine. The two parties do not reach the same feeling, but a consonance of feeling.[16]

Here's an example. Suppose I have received a diagnosis of a virulent, fast-growing cancer. You, as my friend, wish to be in a compassionate relationship to me, so you weep with me, curse Fate and doctors with me, and—with as much imagination as you can—try to feel what I am suffering. I, desiring your friend-ship and consolation and a continuing relationship with you, realize that you cannot fully imagine all that I now experience, so I modulate my feelings to more closely approximate those of which you are capable. It helps, of course, if I am essentially a Calvinist and a Stoic, as Smith was, and if I put a high premium on emotional self-control, or what Smith called "self-command." But what we both desire and aim for is enough accord between our sentiments to continue the friendship; this does not happen automatically, but must be worked for.

The differences between Hume and Smith can be illustrated by the metaphor of the mirror in their works. For Hume, remember, sentiments mirror each other in a continuing, reflective series of reverberations. Sympathy is just this echoing resemblance. By contrast, Smith uses the image of the mirror to indicate how each person breaks out of his natural partiality or self-love. The mirror is society, and through it, or in it, we are enabled to see ourselves. It is the interaction we have in society that empowers us to scru-tinize our own behavior, for only through our social relations can we imagine how our actions look to others.[17] Thus sympathy can be described as the power to duplicate ourselves while at the same time retaining our identity. We become other people, though we remain who we are. This power can also be focused on ourselves, as we view ourselves from the outside, as others see us. In brief, for Hume the mirror is simply a reflecting devise; for Smith it is an instrument for critical examination and dialect-ical exchange.

In rehearsing the moral philosophies of Hume and Smith I have no wish to rehabilitate sympathy per se, or argue for it as a central concept in contemporary ethics. Nor do I wish to argue that Hume and Smith were right in their claim (against the ration-alists) that sentiment (rather than reason) is the foundation of ethics. Neither of these questions can be settled here. Rather, this explication of the notion of sympathy is intended to focus atten-tion on phenomena most persons would recognize as valid: the inherent human affinity for relationships that is denied by social atomism, and the necessity for ethically interdependent relation-ships that is neglected by moral atomism. The precise terms for reference and explication of these phenomena are not important. In his later ethical writings Hume used a variety of terms for sympathy, among them *humanity* and *fellow-feeling*. The terms matter less than the recognition that these indelibly social experiences are the foundation of social cohesiveness, the sharing of benefits and burdens that characterizes solidarity. The twentieth-century French philosopher and psychologist Maurice Merleau-Ponty said it well: "the social is already there when we come to know it or judge it."[18]

Shrinking the *We:* Interest Groups in Health Care

Even those who are fully convinced by Hume and Smith (or their own experience) that social affinity is an indelible aspect of the human situation may be skeptical that it will help us develop a health care system. Such skepticism might seem appropriately to follow from the relative modesty of my claim in this chapter, especially if we leave aside the claims of previous chapters. More specifically, I have argued here that atomism is a faulty picture of self and society, and that a more accurate portrayal must accredit human proclivities for association. I have not argued that universal care will spring from sympathy, only that sympathy can be developed and enhanced in the service of universal care. Sympathy is one sign that the soil to nurture an inclusive system is more fertile than atomistic approaches have led us to believe. If we are to move to an inclusive system, the task we must undertake is not (the Herculean) one of creating a convivial community from a collection of solipsists.

Yet room for skepticism is built into the argument. Simply affirming that persons are essentially social does not necessarily, or even probably, lead to affirmations of universal care; it does not mean that a universal We will develop, especially if smaller and more personal associations already claim our loyalties. Although atomism may be an appealing philosophical and political myth, the more accurate sociological picture is not one of sovereign individuals but of sovereign groups: individuals engaging in selective patterns of association with others on the basis of income, occupation, race, religious orientation, ethnic origin, and other factors. In other words, skepticism may seem to be in order here because the more serious enemy of universal care may not be the solitary I of atomism but the shrunken We of special interests.

Special interest associations are an enduring part of American culture and American politics, and they are not necessarily negative forces. Yet in health care they have tended to be divisive, to act according to the definition James Madison offered for a faction: "a number of citizens, whether amounting to a majority or minority of the whole, who are united and actuated by some common impulse or passion, or of interest, adverse to the rights of other citizens, or to the permanent and aggregate interests of the community."[19]

Hume was keenly aware of the problems of factionalism. Religious zealotry, and the long and bloody history of Europe's religious wars, received his greatest condemnation as a destructive force disrupting civil society. He believed that the tendency toward animosity based on differences both real and imaginary, both significant and trivial, was an enduring, dark side of human nature. Moreover, he saw that these antipathies frequently continue even after the original reasons for the dispute have disappeared.

> Nothing is more usual than to see parties, which have begun upon a real difference, continue even after that difference is lost. When men are once enlisted on opposite sides, they contract an affection to the persons with whom they are united, and an animosity against their antagonists; and these passions they often transmit to their posterity.[20]

For Hume, the hot passions of parochial interests—locally identified and reinforced in exclusive associations of "us" and "them"—are a constant threat to the reflective, prudential calculations that relate personal to social goods.

Derek Phillips has recently argued an even stronger thesis in asserting that communitarian politics of the common good almost always turn out to be associations of "us" set off to dominate an excluded "them." Arguing from a study of the particulars (rather than the republican rhetoric) of ancient Athens and colonial America, Phillips says: "the moral thrust of the communitarian ideal . . . is simultaneously to unite and divide . . . For the attempt to realize community not only requires a strong sense of solidarity and belonging but also seems to require the presence of enemies within and without."[21] According to Phillips the banner of the "common good" is most frequently a screen behind which special interests can be pursued. The dark side of solidarity is its tendency to exclude, morally judge, and dominate others—

all under the ideology of communitarian virtues and the common good.

Although he does not have health care in mind, Phillips's thesis underscores my argument for universal care. A solidarity that is less than inclusive not only thwarts self-interest but threatens to become politically tyrannical and morally abusive. Phillips's arguments also confirm the strategies I have used in this volume—namely, to refuse to make assumptions of communitarian benevolence the foundations for health care, and, instead, to make a rational, inclusive solidarity an aim of the system, enhanced by (but not founded on) benevolent motives.

In health care the selective and restricted We is a persistent hazard on the road to a universal solidarity. The current fragmented approach to providing and financing services both creates and reinforces divisions. It tends to pit the insured against the uninsured, payers against "free riders," cancer or heart disease programs against AIDS programs, the needs of the elderly against the needs of children, and perhaps most damaging, the interests of providers against the needs of uninsured patients. Factious elements are present and powerful, and they will no doubt continue to influence health policy. So the skeptic is correct in doubting whether a simple affirmation of social affinities can reduce interest group divisiveness or bring about a more inclusive We in health care.

My answer to the skeptic is to return her attention to the first three chapters. The skepticism that may arise here cannot be rebutted by appeals to sympathy, but rather by reference to the power of rational self-interest in the context of four factors already discussed: (1) the scarcity of health resources relative to health problems; (2) the uncontrolled growth in health care expenditures; (3) the largely unpredictable nature of health care needs; and, above all, (4) the precarious nature of anyone's status as "insured." The skeptic should reread Chapter 3 for the case against factions in health care, that is, for the reasons that an exclusive or restricted solidarity ultimately serves no one. She will be convinced there, or not at all. If she is convinced, universal solidarity should seem a more lively possibility after atomism is discredited. If she is not, further exhibits of our affinity for association will not convince her.

CHAPTER FIVE

Rights and Responsibilities: Health Care Goals and Moral Coherence

Espousing security and solidarity does not necessarily lead to affirmation of a right to health care. Other countries that provide basic health services to all citizens have found ways to interpret their aims without relying heavily on rights language. Enthusiasm for rights—and the use of rights language to cover large areas of personal and political life—may well be an American peculiarity, stemming from our recent beginnings in revolution and the desire to protect the freedoms of individuals from tyrannical governments. It could be argued that cashing out the aims of a health care system in terms of an individual entitlement will do more harm than good. Federal entitlement programs are frequently associated with escalating costs and with interest group politics and may actually thwart the realization of security and solidarity. A decade ago the President's Commission for the Study of Ethical Problems in Medicine and Biomedical and Behavioral Research carefully avoided speaking of access to health care as a right, preferring to say instead that "society has an ethical obligation to ensure equitable access to health care for all."[1] Using rights to set the framework for health care reform at least initially leads away from the goals I have embraced, and it may lead to a set of priorities in which entitlements are understood as private possessions rather than as expressions of personal security in the context of social solidarity.

Yet despite these cautionary notes it seems desirable to talk about the goals of health care in terms of rights. One reason is practical. Rights language about health care is already a lively part of the national debate. In his 1991 State of the Union address, George Bush endorsed a right to health care, even though the extent of that right was largely unspecified. In the 1992 elections, the Democratic Party platform advocated a right to health care. For Americans health ranks above wealth and personal achievement as "the greatest single source of happiness."[2] Nine out of ten persons polled in 1987 said that "everybody should have the right to get the best possible health care—as good as the treatment a millionaire gets."[3] For better or worse, a right to health care seems embedded in the American vocabulary, and dislodging it may not be possible.

In addition, there are morally important reasons to retain rights language. First, to speak of access to health care as a right signals the critical importance of health services in gaining and retaining opportunity to the other goods and goals of life. This central instrumental value of health care can be reflected by calling it a right. Speaking of a social obligation, in the absence of a clearly understood individual entitlement, simply does not carry the same weight. Second, a right to health services implies that access to care need not be justified on utilitarian grounds. My right of access to basic services, for example to a primary care physician, need not satisfy a "greatest good for the greatest number" test. Such access should be securely and unalienably mine; it may be circumscribed by constrained resources, but it should not be overridden by considerations of utility. Third, a right to health care is empowering; it obligates government to make provision for whatever level of services is specified in the right, thus enhancing security. Finally, rights language bespeaks a basic equality, enfranchising the politically weak and the sick; it renders irrelevant differences in health status, income, age, race, gender, and other social characteristics. It thereby works in the service of inclusiveness and solidarity. So despite the caveats listed above, the goals of security and solidarity are congenial to rights language and are perhaps best understood in this way.

Rights language should not, however, be the point of entry into the policy debate. It is too laden with adversarial connotations to work well as the centerpiece of reform, and it should not set the framework for discussion. It should appear as it does in this volume, near the end, and as a way of making more concrete and giving focus to the overall goals. When properly articulated as an expression of these larger aims, a right to health care services is a very useful concept. It is to that proper articulation that I now turn.

If health care is to become a *tangible* right in the United States, and not merely a hortatory ideal, a way must be found to define the scope of that right. A system of health care that entitled all citizens to all possible services would be financially infeasible. We currently spend more than 14 percent of our Gross Domestic Product (GDP) on health care, yet 25 percent of the population is unserved or underserved. If we were to provide health coverage to everyone and leave other aspects of the system unchanged, health expenditures would immediately consume 20 percent of the GDP and continue to escalate. No one believes this is economically possible, let alone desirable. Hence, greater equity in coverage can be achieved only if ways can be found to limit health care services and reform the financing and delivery of these services.

In a previous work I sought to articulate a working principle for a right to health care, that is, a principle that affirms access to care as fundamental yet also recognizes that there are limits to the level and kind of services to which any person can be entitled.[4] Need, I argued, is the essential criterion for access: need cannot be superseded by financial, social worth, or other considerations. But not all needs can be met, and in the United States our seemingly insatiable appetite for health services means than desires for higher levels of well-being or for reassurance quickly turn into needs. So a full rendering of a right to care must contain provisions for parsimony in defining access and need. A right to health care based on need means, then, a right to equitable access based on need alone to all effective care society can reasonably afford.

The term *equity* is used to signal proportionality, as opposed to sheer numerical, equality. Because needs vary among people—often dramatically—a policy of strictly equal access would not be equitable.

My call for equity "based on need alone" is intended to signal the morally arbitrary nature of race, gender, income, and other differences as criteria for access to care. Any given person's needs are equivalent to anyone else's. No one holds a prior place in the health care queue because of social worth or wealth. Whatever hierarchy of needs is devised to distribute services cannot be calculated to privilege persons because of their social or financial power.

The term *effective care* calls into play an essential limiting device. It is intended to curtail useless treatments and duplicative testing, and also to substantially curb high-tech interventions of marginal utility. Making this criterion work would require a much greater degree of professional consensus than we now enjoy about what services are truly important, not to mention a way of reducing so-called defensive medicine through malpractice reforms. Consensus and reform in these areas will be a necessary part of any proposal that hopes to contain costs, not just mine.

Finally, by specifying "what society can reasonably afford" I am acknowledging that some pressing needs in health care will inevitably not be met. No modern society anywhere has devised a way to meet all the health needs of its population, even if we exclude those marginally effective services that some would insist are necessary. Needs will always outrun the ability to meet them. Unless we are willing to cripple or eliminate other social programs, health care must be limited in a prudent balancing of health services with education, housing, social services, highways, and dozens of others. This necessary restriction on the extent of services provided does not, however, mitigate the idea of a right to some level of services. As Tom Beauchamp and Ruth Faden have put it, a right to health care is unalienable (it cannot be taken away) but not absolute. It can be overridden by other social priorities and is always contingent on the amount of resources society is prepared to allot to the provision of health services.[5]

In brief, the recognition of limits to the right of access—limits that can be affirmed as fair—is pivotal. Without some realistic and morally coherent notion of limits, all talk of a right to health care is utopian. A variety of ways to limit services can be imagined—by a person's age, by the effectiveness of services, by their cost, and so on. Yet to specify criteria for limiting services jumps a critical step in the process. It seeks detail in the absence of a general moral warrant. Absent this moral warrant, most persons might agree in principle that there must be limits but few would feel obligated to accept them, especially for programs that directly affect them or their families. We cannot talk about limiting programs for the elderly, or for the terminally ill, or for anyone, until we have first talked about limits as a moral, and not just an economic, concept. Scarcity and cost underwrite the limitation on health services economically, but to make limits morally coherent will require a notion of responsibility to complement a right to health services.

In what follows I will examine two ways of aligning rights and responsibilities, a Response Model and a Good Behavior Model.[6] These are only two of many possible ways to consider the issue, but examining these two ways will help clarify the values involved.

The Good Behavior Model

Rights have corresponding responsibilities. For example, the right to freedom of expression entails a corresponding duty not to slander or defame. This marks the limits of free speech and makes it socially viable as a right. In a similar fashion, it is the exercise of responsibility that makes a right to health care viable. Often that responsibility in health care is conceived as a responsibility for good health practices. Here the logic of responsibility holds that accountability for one's own health is justified by what we know about the effects of individual life-style choices on health status. I will call this way of thinking the Good Behavior Model, because it implies that the right to health services is forfeited, or at least weakened, if one indulges in behavior harmful to health.

The attraction in this way of thinking is obvious. Individuals clearly do have some control over their own health status and their need for medical services. The extent of this control, it is argued, should mark the extent of individual responsibility. Many illnesses and injuries are seen as "self-inflicted," through bad habits. Smoking, excessive alcohol consumption, overeating, and high-cholesterol-and-low-fiber diets are only a few of the examples. Driving without seat belts, riding a motorcycle without a helmet, and engaging in unprotected sexual activity are others. The problems that may result—lung cancer, emphysema, cirrhosis of the liver, coronary artery disease, gastrointestinal cancers, motor vehicle injuries and fatalities, and a variety of sexually transmitted diseases—are perceived as having been caused by choosing to live in an unhealthy way. Such diseases add both to societal ill health and to health care expenditures.

In the Good Behavior Model, smokers, for example, would have a lesser right to treatment for lung cancer than nonsmokers enjoy. They might lose their claim to these resources altogether. Alcoholics would relinquish any claim to liver transplants, helmetless motorcycle riders would have diminished access to emergency medical services, drug abusers to coronary care units, and so on.

This sort of thinking received a substantial boost in 1991 from the then Secretary of Health and Human Services, Dr. Louis W. Sullivan. In his "Foreword" to *Healthy People 2000*—the U.S. Public Health Service document that was intended to set "the Nation's disease prevention and health promotion agenda for this decade"—Dr. Sullivan endorsed the Good Behavior Model in its causal form, and thereby aided those who would endorse it as a criterion for access to care, or as a criterion for payment for care received.

Sullivan's basic point was that "personal responsibility, responsible and enlightened behavior by each and every individual, truly is the key to good health."[7] He followed this claim with a litany of the health hazards of smoking, alcohol, and drug abuse and the benefits of fitness and good nutrition. Asserting that "we can control our health destinies in significant ways," Sullivan finally endorsed what he called a "culture of character," namely, a way of thinking and acting that would reflect responsible health practices. Building this "culture of character," he contended, was "an absolute necessity."

There is no question that Sullivan is correct, but to a far more limited extent than his rhetoric suggested. Yet the problem is not so much his inflated statements about the range of personal control over our health destinies. The more serious pitfall in his thinking is signaled by his use of moralizing language. Health problems, he says, result from deficient "character," from lack of responsibility for one's health habits. To be sure, he does not argue for good character as a criterion for access to care, but all that he says lends credibility to this practice. To single out the personal responsibility of individuals is, of course, to deflect attention away from governmental inaction and professional neglect of the "irresponsible" sick, especially if they are uninsured. The language of individual moral faultfinding is a favorite idiom used to conceal ineptness in social policy in many realms. But the central point is that Sullivan invites us to embrace a logic that begins rather innocently in good behavior yet threatens to end in denial of care for the impoverished sick because of their profligate behavior. It is a short step from the premise of a "culture of character," implying that the ill have created their own health problems, to the conclusion that therefore they do not merit treatment. A "culture of character" is easily correlated with inaction toward (and moralistic advice for) the "undeserving sick."

A central problem with the Good Behavior Model is its exaggerated notion of control. While it has its roots in the American reverence for self-reliance and individual responsibility, control over one's health status and the extent of one's need for medical services is far from complete. Some behavioral factors in ill health may be only partially voluntary—for example, addiction to cigarettes, alcohol, or controlled substances. Other behavioral risks are embedded in cultural dietary traditions, or in poor nutrition, or in living and working environments highly associated with socio-economic status. An individual's responsibility cannot exceed his or her ability to choose.

Efforts to base access to health care (or payment for health services) on individual responsibility for one's health status are suspect and should be avoided. Such efforts frequently exaggerate our knowledge of causes or ignore multiple factors in the causes of diseases. They also run the risk of blaming the victim. Dan Beauchamp puts it eloquently: "Victim-blaming misdefines structural and collective problems of the entire society as individual problems, seeing these problems as caused by the behavioral failures or deficiencies of the victims."[8]

In sum, the Good Behavior Model tends to be an instrument for disenfranchising persons rather than enabling them. It separates a class of individuals from their peers and associates, often through a flawed and simplistic notion of causation, and, in the worst cases, it stigmatizes those who are likely to need medical assistance the most. As a way of conceptualizing responsibility, this model threatens to undermine the security of persons for access to and payment for health services. Because it places limits on services in a way that tends to judge persons morally, it is essentially a segregation by social worth. It cannot serve the larger goal of solidarity.

Responsibility for one's health status should, of course, be the focus of substantial educational and public health efforts. Active promotion of healthy life-styles and sound health habits is altogether laudatory. Yet to step beyond this educational mission and "scold" people for their behavioral flaws is dangerous. Responsibility for individual health-related behaviors is only one dimension of a just overall health policy. If taken by itself, and as way of curtailing rights to services, it will lead us in the wrong direction.

The Response Model

In the face of limited health care resources, the key responsibility for the individual is to have realistic expectations and to make wise use of these resources. It is the obligation of every one of us to think of health care services not only as a private benefit but as a social and public good as well.

This connection can be called the Response Model of linking rights and responsibilities. Rights to health care are provided by a society, and in response the individual takes responsibility for using only his or her fair share. The response of taking only a fair share should not be understood as a response of gratitude. The provision of health services is not a gift. Gifts require grateful behavior from the recipients, and the logic of gifts and gratitude is very different from that of rights and responsibilities. For example, no one need be grateful for having his right to free speech respected. It is simply what is due. Yet persons who exercise free speech do so within social boundaries that protect others from slander and defamation. In a similar way, any workable right to health care must have similar boundaries. I call this the Response Model to indicate that a response (not of gratitude, but of fair and judicious use) is required. It is important to see the recipient's attitude to health care as a response, and not just an acceptance, because self-conscious activity is called for. Medical services cannot be taken for granted, for it is the parsimony of personal privilege in using health resources that allows the system to remain viable, both for oneself and for others.

The Response Model is attuned to the goal of solidarity. It entails assent to the idea that a health care system must be largely shaped and defined by the health needs of the population rather than the personal needs and preferences of the most powerful interest groups. In many countries, this means tolerating a waiting period for some nonemergency treatments and accepting that services may be denied if they satisfy personal desires but have little or no bearing on the health status of individuals or the population. Examples include cosmetic procedures, excessive diagnostic tests that offer reassurance, and expensive treatments of marginal utility near the end of life.

For example, in Canada and the United Kingdom the supply of hospitals, surgeons, and intensive care units is limited, so there are fewer solid organ transplants. There are waiting periods for elective surgeries, such as hip replacements, and a limited supply of money and facilities for CT scanners. There is less aggressive chemotherapy and radiation treatment for advanced cancer. Yet all citizens of both countries are provided access to a primary care physician, and their general health status is as good as or better than that of U.S. citizens. Ultimately, deciding which health services to provide and which to forgo is a public policy question. The point is that in *any* system, some services will have to be limited if there is to be equity of access and proportionate funding left for schools, roads, defense, and the like.

A viable and fair health care system is a "public good" in which all citizens have a stake. All share a common human vulnerability to disease, disability, and death. All of us face the future without knowing when or how urgently we will need health services. We all support through tax dollars the creation and maintenance of the various institutions of health care, including hospitals, and the education of health professionals. All have a stake in a healthy populace above and beyond the stake each has in his or her personal health. And, as I have argued, all have an interest in making provision for care universal, rather than partial.

These shared interests point to a shared responsibility for ensuring the judicious use of the resources that we possess. The responsibility individuals have is not only or primarily for choosing our own life-styles but for controlling our general expectations of a system that is understood to be finite. ⊄

Individuals will assume responsibility for using and supporting a health care system only when that system is seen to be equitable and just. In short, this health-related civic responsibility will never evolve without a general right of access to adequate health care for all. The current patchwork system that allocates health services by price, by age, and by employment status, and leaves a quarter of the population underinsured or uninsured, cannot inspire a sense of responsibility, either individual or collective. Our current system takes a consumer-oriented approach to health care, one that encourages us to satisfy all our personal health needs regardless of the effect this has on the well-being of others. Not only is this approach disrespectful of others, it is ultimately self-defeating.

Defining One's Fair Share

If the Response Model of aligning rights and responsibilities means that every person should be prepared to use only a fair share of the resources, then it becomes important how a fair share is defined. Does this mean, for example, that a person faced with a life-threatening illness should forgo expensive treatments? Or that when making such a decision for a family member we should begin to think of the equitable distribution of resources across society before seeking treatment? A purely quantitative notion of a share might mean that each person is eligible to receive, for example, up to (and no more than) $500,000 worth of care. Here a share would function like a maximum benefit in a conventional indemnity health insurance policy. Yet these ways of conceiving of a fair share obscure the point by taking tertiary care as the normative perspective and by considering purely quantitative notions of shares.

Expecting everyone to calculate shares on the way to the hospital would be an impossibly high requirement, and probably morally perverse. It would subvert our most powerful obligations—those to ourselves and to our families. But this does not mean that the fair share is an unworkable idea. Rather, the mis-take is in thinking of shares as pieces of a pie that are parceled out in an ad hoc fashion to individuals who are at the point of extreme hunger or starvation. A share is not a quantifiable unit of services, or a dollar maximum allotted to individuals, but a way of underscoring the scarcity of a resource created by the public and intended for common use.

The central idea of shares is *sharing* a resource, not making claim to a unit of services as though they were subject to private ownership. The private property notion of a share subverts the notion of sharing, or holding in common. My "fair share" is not my personal, disposable unit; it is the way I must think about my role in creating and using the resources for health that are available.

The design of a new system of health care must be fair in its inception and devise policies of allotting resources across society as a whole. Fairness does not suddenly arise in life-and-death scenarios. In the absence of a fair system, considerations of fairness cannot emerge as an element in individual decision-making about care, as we saw earlier in reference to age-rationing.

An emphasis on an individual's "fair share" will not, of course, eliminate problems with regard to how many services physicians should offer or patients should ask for in difficult cases. It should, however, change the focus from a case-by-case reaction to a policy approach. Instead of deciding on an ad hoc basis which persons to admit to the Intensive Care Unit, we should decide how many Intensive Care Units there will be, where they will be located, and the guidelines for their use. Fairness in decisions at the individual level depends upon the context provided by a fair system overall.

In summary, developing a viable and fair health care system does not mean simply providing coverage for the medically indigent, important as that is. Given the escalating costs of health care, more of the same for more people is a recipe for economic disaster. Reforms to the system in financing and organization are essential, but even they are not sufficient. Financial and organizational reforms must be preceded by reforms in our thinking.

One such critical reform is linking a right to health care services with responsible use of those services, while avoiding the erroneous and punitive Good Behavior Model. The notion that a right has to be earned by good behavior, as this forfeiture model portrays it, undermines its status as a right and makes it ultimately a commodity granted to the behaviorally worthy. A health care system based on rewards for good behavior would be just as morally flawed as one that granted a right to health care on the basis of race or gender. The Good Behavior Model, in sum, focuses on the grounds for disqualification, whereas the Response Model focuses on the civic virtues appropriate to participation in the system.

The Response Model allows us to talk of health care as a social good, and not just as an individual good, because the response of judicious use and acceptance of limits is a response to a social policy of fairness. It opens the way for a noncommercial concept of health care as part of the social and public world—the world which we all hold in common. This concept can be further clarified by recasting rights and responsibilities in civic terms and thinking of both patients and physicians as citizens.[9]

Citizenship for Doctors and Patients

A citizen is considered a member of a state who owes allegiance to a (justly constituted) government and is entitled to protection from it. The liberal, personal side of citizenship emphasizes the legal status of individual members as defined by both negative rights and positive entitlements. In this understanding, citizenship is seen as a shell of protection for the underlying private self. The communitarian side of citizenship emphasizes common purposes and shared vulnerabilities among the individual members. This latter understanding of citizenship identifies the self as essentially social, as constituted by civic relationships, and emphasizes responsibility to those relationships. Both facets of citizenship are important to the ethics of health care. In contemporary analyses, the more private and individual facet has dominated. I will emphasize here the social aspect of citizenship in order to balance the discussion. Any workable ethic for health care will need to acknowledge the importance of both dimensions.

Citizenship evokes a sense of belonging to something larger than self, something greater than particular individual relationships. "Citizens" of a health care system are persons whose allegiances extend beyond private interests and beyond patient-specific professional duties to a sociopolitical order. Citizens both enjoy the rights and protections of that order and incur responsibilities for its maintenance and well-being. Persons with health problems are not only patients with rights but citizens with duties. The right of access to services and to make health care decisions should not be seen as absolutes without a context but as liberties bounded by the limited resources of society and the parallel rights of others.

Traditionally, the patient has been seen as a powerless dependent. Talcott Parson's classic definition of the "sick role" was for many years the paradigm for patient behavior—dependence, passivity, and compliance with doctor's orders combined with a pervasive desire to recover.[10] Progress in medical ethics over the past two decades can in part be measured by the extent to which more active and morally enfranchised roles for patients have developed. Concepts such as the patient as person and patients' rights have become common currency. When taken alone, however, the notion of patients' rights is too narrow, and responsibilities that accompany the granting of rights are infrequently affirmed and not widely recognized.[11] The idea of patients as citizens can help to bring these responsibilities to the foreground and give a civic context to the notion of restraint.

Restraint in the use of health resources is certainly not a new idea. Norman Daniels, as we have seen, believes that proportionate rationing of the use of health resources would be the sort of "prudent" choices made by hypothetical "rational agents" who allocate fair shares of basic social goods over a lifetime.[12] The "Prudential Lifespan Account" supports restrictions on some medical care at the end of life and favors more intergenerational equity than we have at present. Daniel Callahan, as noted in Chapter 1, argues for much the same goal in a different vein, claiming that our present all-out efforts to extend life at the edges are contrary to the purposes of medicine and prohibit attention to the true needs of the elderly for a more independent and financially secure life.[13]

The novel aspect of my thesis is the contention that citizenship can provide a moral glue, an ethical coherence, for thinking about how to participate in a health care system. The motivation for judiciously restrained use of resources is best expressed as a civic one. Were we all "rational agents" or "life planners" ignorant of our particular histories, or were we endowed with greater general benevolence, civic motivation would perhaps be unnecessary. But we are not. Defining our participation in the health system as citizenship is one way (though not the only way) to more fittingly address the realities of our situation, to affirm both rights and responsibilities, and to achieve both personal security and social solidarity.

Citizenship should be carefully distinguished from the religious aspects of stewardship. For example, in Christian doctrine stewardship refers to the use of God's gifts. Stewards are given possessions "in trust," and the possessions with which they are entrusted are never unequivocally theirs. They are, rather, held for use in accord with Providential purposes. By contrast, citizens can claim rights to which they are unequivocally entitled. Also, the responsibilities of citizenship are not transcendentally fixed but socially shaped. A purely secular interpretation of stewardship—an individual's responsibility to manage his life and property with proper regard to the rights of others—expresses well the central point I wish to emphasize.

If all patients have obligations as citizens, then all citizens must have access to the rights of patienthood. If individuals can be asked to assume social duties, even when ill, it will be because all ill citizens can first be recognized as having a fundamental right to adequate or basic care. Without this umbrella of societal inclusion for all the sick, no patient would be motivated by the responsibilities of citizenship to conserve resources. When only the upper classes have rights, each decision to forgo care at the margins is idiosyncratic, a gesture of altruism or particular beliefs. A societal decision to include all persons in health care services serves as the backdrop against which proportionate choices can be seen as the usual duties of common citizenship. Choices to forgo marginal care can become forces for social cohesion, if they can draw at least a part of their authority from a public policy that extends access to health care benefits to all. Responsibilities *within* health care can then be seen as abiding in a context of rights *to* health care, with each modifying the other.

The physician must also be seen as a citizen. Historically, medical oaths, codes, and principles of ethics have recognized a variety of allegiances in addition to the physician's allegiance to the patient. The Oath of Hippocrates invokes the sanction of divine authorities and pledges fidelity to teachers, colleagues, and students. Medieval expressions of duty, such as the Prayer of Maimonides, place obligations to patients in the larger context of religious responsibilities. The American Medical Association's most recent "Principles of Medical Ethics," dating from 1980, lists responsibilities not only to patients "but also to society, to other health professionals and to self."[14]

Citizenship as a source of moral obligation for physicians is noted explicitly in the AMA's first official effort to define its responsibilities, the Code of 1847. Chapter 3, article 1 of the Code begins in the following way: "As good citizens, it is the duty of physicians to be ever vigilant for the welfare of the community and to bear their part in sustaining its institutions and burdens."[15] The authors of this code conceived as citizen duties such matters as advice on hygiene, quarantine regulations, the management of epidemics, and the location of hospitals, not the fair distribution of medical manpower or resource allocation. Yet the concept of citizenship as a moral component of medical ethics was recognized and presumably accepted by the profession. So the idea of citizenship as a source of medical obligations is not new. What is new is the contention that citizenship should play a different and larger role than in the past. A larger role is required because of the differences between American medical care in the mid-nineteenth and the late twentieth century.

If medical care were only marginally effective or of questionable value in preserving life and restoring health, physicians' responsibilities of citizenship could be carefully circumscribed, as in 1847, to matters of hygiene and quarantine. When, however, medical care becomes effective enough to be a socially recognized need, and as soon as society invests substantially in its provision from public funds, the responsibilities of physicians as citizens must be enlarged. Medical care is no longer a privately bought, individual good of marginal value; it now has the status of a largely public-supported individual and social good of great benefit. Some believe medical care is in fact overvalued. Yet even if there is debate about its value, or what constitutes an appropriate amount of care, few would disagree that at least a basic provision of care is essential to a decent life.

With this increase in value comes an increase in the importance of a citizenship component in medical ethics. Michael Walzer puts it succinctly: "Doctors and hospitals have become such massively important features of contemporary life that to be cut off from the help they provide is not only dangerous but also degrading."[16] In other words, the rationale for calling for a greater citizen ethic for physicians is at least partially grounded in the need in any democracy to preserve the self-respect of citizens.

Many of my physician colleagues who know first-hand the importance of placing limits on health care spending have difficulty with the idea that patients and doctors have social duties in health care relationships and not just personal and professional ones. "Society should set the limits," they say, "and we'll live within them," hoping thereby to keep the professional realm hermetically sealed from social influences. In general it does seem both wise and necessary for major policy decisions to be made at a remove from the bedside. Yet no set of policies, however well conceived, can encompass the diverse range of choices involved in medical care. Nor does it seem wise to restrict clinical judgment in this way. But the more important point is that no policy will be feasible unless it has moral cogency, unless it makes sense to both patients and physicians in their roles as patients and physicians. To speak of patients and physicians as citizens invokes that cogency; it focuses on the civic moral authority necessary for any health care system to work. Social responsibilities are not, then, vague, bureaucratic requirements imposed upon a private relationship, but the civic duties of doctors and patients in the context of therapeutic encounters.

It might be thought that a citizen ethic will weaken the physician's ability to assist patients in need because of state or bureaucratic controls on the practice of medicine. Just the opposite is more likely. The current reactive system of health care financing hampers continuity of the patient-physician relationship and results in sporadic care and extreme fluctuations in access. A rationalized and more efficient system, combined with a citizen ethic of judicious use, would eliminate the need to micromanage physicians through utilization reviews and cost-accounting of thousands of separate procedures. Within accepted policy limitations, physicians should enjoy a greater degree of freedom in clinical judgment and patients should enjoy greater continuity of care.

Some may object that a physician-patient relationship that includes an element of common citizen obligations will make the therapeutic alliance less private or confidential. Yet a citizen ethic does not subject doctor-patient encounters to public scrutiny. It simply means that the limits on what therapies can be offered have a larger social sanction than they have now, as artifacts of employability, commercial forces of distribution, institutional or professional largesse, or idiosyncratic entitlements. To be sure, some limits on the marginal benefits that patients can expect to receive or physicians can offer will be necessary, but this will not drive a wedge into the patient-physician relationship. It will provide both physicians and patients a common allegiance in addition to the separate motives both parties now bring to the therapeutic encounter.

Finally, it may be thought that the sort of restraint implied in a citizen ethic will require supererogatory acts of individual patients, forgoing care they believe they are entitled to in order to benefit others. Yet to think of restrained choices as supererogatory, or above and beyond the call of duty, bespeaks an assumption of an unlimited right to services. It is precisely this unbounded sense of entitlement that has caused some of the problems we now face. Choosing health care services with restraint should be understood as the ordinary and routine obligation everyone incurs in order for the health care system to work.

In summary, a citizen ethic in health care is not just a way for physicians to say no to patients who may want more services than can justly be offered to them. It is also a way to understand the inevitable no's that must be said, at both the individual and the policy level. The unavailability of a service that patients might want can become morally coherent if patients see themselves and their physicians as citizens participating fairly in a system that is just, but limited. As Daniels has argued, in the current arrangements physicians have difficulty saying no to any patient inside the clinic or hospital walls because—in the absence of a rational and just system—every no seems arbitrary, an unanchored and groundless denial.[17] And while a denial is contextless for physicians and patients intramurally, a wholesale rejection is tacitly transmitted to those outside the walls who lack the admissions credentials of money or insurance. By contrast, citizenship imbeds the yes's and no's of health care in civic rights and responsibilities, where they support the goals of security and solidarity. In Humean terms, a citizen ethic is the means by which the "common sense of interest" can be "mutually express'd."

A Concluding Image:

Voices of Reciprocity

The "common sense of interest" of which Hume spoke can be thought of in various ways. He spoke directly about a self-interest that is "common" to humans, meaning experienced by everyone. To turn the meaning a bit, Hume's approach is also "common sense," meaning commonplace or ordinary, not hypothetical or sophisticated. It does not rely on philosophical speculation or great feats of imagination, but appeals instead to lived experiences that he believed every reflective person would recognize. Still, this reliance on common experiences and common sense does not mean that one can arrive at justice automatically or easily.

The metaphor of the vault, as discussed in Chapter 3, with its interlocking and mutually supportive pieces, is a good image for the structural components of justice. Yet, if taken as an image of the social dynamics of interdependence, it lacks a central element. Arrangements for security, Hume thought, would develop more or less naturally from reflection about our private self-interests. But this common sense of interest in a secure life leads to just institutions only when it is "mutually express'd." The element missing in the image of the vault is self-conscious expression of the commonly recognized need.

I argued in Chapter 5 that citizenship is a concept that can serve us well in articulating this commonly recognized need. Health policy should engage us as public and civic persons, not simply appeal to us as private and individuated consumers. Yet a full and convincing expression of this commonly recognized self-interest for universal care will likely take many years to come about. Health care reform proposals, focusing largely on economic and organizational matters, will not contain all the ethical language we will need to express a new and more just social compact. Nor could they. One of the lessons of Hume is that the language of the common weal cannot be simply created intellectually, or as a preamble to a just system; it must be forged through the efforts to make a just system work. It is the practices of just health care—and critical reflection on those practices—that will, finally, provide us with a fully adequate way to speak. The important thing at this juncture is to start, to give some expression, however provisional, to the morally important features of universal care.

This concluding chapter is an effort to give voice to our acknowledged interdependence—to an image of how we must begin to think and talk about our self-interest and our common interest in the context of health care system goals. This image is designed to keep before us the fact that justice is possible only when the common interest can be made visible. It is designed to highlight a picture of health behaviors and choices in which exchange, interdependence, and mutual regard are prominent. It should also assist in developing mental habits that situate the I in a We context, that give voice to the civic self in health care situations.

Imagine I have a headache of one week's duration. The pain is not intense, but it is relatively constant, and it is only partially relieved by the usual over-the-counter medications. I visit a physician who obtains a brief history and does an abbreviated physical examination, which yields no significant findings. The physician tells me the cause of my headache is likely stress, allergies, or some self-limiting condition of unknown origin. At this point I might suggest a CT scan, or even an MRI, or a referral to a specialist. If my anxiety is high enough, I could revise my history to exaggerate my symptoms and thereby smooth the passage for additional tests or a referral. What I seek is a higher level of reassurance that I do not have a brain tumor or some other catastrophic disease.

Most of us (well-insured "consumers" of health services) have been schooled to think we should ask how the system can better serve our needs and wants. So we are prone to approach this situation asking what services we would ideally desire for ourselves. Yet, as I have argued, asking about our health in an idealized way jeopardizes everyone's security. If we are to achieve security and solidarity, we must recognize that the voice that expresses idealized assumptions about health and well-being is dysfunctional.

Justice requires that the voice expressing my health care needs and wants must be a responsive one, as discussed earlier. What would that mean here? It would mean that I must frame my choices and behaviors in a way that acknowledges the reciprocity of standard-setting among myself and all others who use the system. It means that I must be willing for others to receive, from public resources, that level of services I consider appropriate for myself; and whatever I will for others to have should also set the limits for my own use. So in making choices for myself, I set the standard for others, and they do the same for me as they choose. It is in this sense that the dominant picture of health-seeking behaviors must be both responsive (to the granting of a right of access) and reciprocal (an exchange of standard-setting values and priorities with others).

My health care appetites can then be exercised with greater parsimony, because I recognize that they will become standards for universal care. My tendency to disregard or neglect the needs of others is, then, tempered by my recognition that I can receive from public resources only what others will for me to receive through their choices. An exercise in this kind of reciprocal entitlement has the appeal of concreteness and a directly felt exchange. The key issue in reciprocity is not one of hypothetical fairness, or theoretical equity, but one of establishing, in practical terms, what we can all reasonably live with. The setting of standards of care, or services to be made available in a universal package, is, of course, a complex task. I do not suggest that thinking of reciprocal limits is the only element in establishing standards, but it is a key element in making standards morally coherent.

The language of reciprocity does not specify a precise course of action here, but it does frame my thinking about what I am willing to accept in terms of what I am willing for others to have when they are in my situation. Of course, I may feel that all who find themselves in my situation should have access to a CT scan, that is, to (what will very likely be) a slightly higher level of reassurance. But if I choose this course I must also recognize that this use of resources will decrease resources needed to treat or reassure me in other situations, or that it will increase my insurance premiums, or my taxes for health care. The position I cannot assume is one of personal exemption from the general limitations upon resources. I cannot assume I should be able to command the reassurance of sophisticated diagnostic tests while endorsing only verbal reassurance for others.

I have chosen a routine example involving primary care purposefully. Many discussions of health care reform that stress limitations and rationing focus on expensive practices, such as solid organ transplants or the treatment of very low birth weight babies. No doubt, savings will be achieved by reducing the number of high-technology procedures, especially those of limited value. Yet to focus the question of limitations on the most expensive settings may give the impression that primary care practices, and typical American health behaviors, can be left unexamined. Such a focus may also imply that the savings that a new system must ensure can all be garnered from those practices used only in extreme cases and that restraints and limits will not affect us. True health care reform will require a critical look at all aspects of the financing and delivery of health services, and a truly just system will require rethinking the meaning and importance of health services at every physician-patient interface. Indeed, it may turn out that cost containment can only be achieved by de-mythologizing medicine more generally, and by reducing our routine dependence on personal medical services for a meaningful, satisfying life.

In a recent review of Clinton's Health Security Act, Ronald Dworkin has suggested another way to introduce prudence into health care.[1] Dworkin argues—correctly, I believe—that the "rescue principle" has created havoc with our understanding of the importance of health care when compared with other uses of our resources.[2] The rescue principle demands that society provide all possible treatment whenever there is even a remote chance that a life can be saved. Dworkin contends that this mandate results in an unfair system, in the sense that it produces a system of enormous inequity in which some are overtreated while others are left out entirely or receive care too late.

Dworkin's "prudent insurance principle" would balance the anticipated value of medical treatment against other goods and other risks in life. Dworkin believes that most prudent insurers could agree on a benefits package, choosing, for example, to not insure themselves for very expensive and low-benefit bowel and liver transplants while opting for earlier screening for breast or prostate cancer. Whatever services prudent insurers might select, Dworkin argues, their choices would constitute a fair system and should become the standard adopted by Clinton's National Health Board.

I find Dworkin's notion of the ideal prudent purchaser of insurance very helpful, but not as convincing as the Humean approach I have developed in the preceding chapters. My chief objection is that the "prudent purchaser" ideal is *too much* of an ideal. Like other approaches that rely on hypothetical choices, Dworkin's model requires visionary conditions, which he enumerates as: (1) a nearly equal distribution of wealth and income in society; (2) universal and state-of-the-art knowledge about the effectiveness of medical interventions; and (3) ignorance about an individual's personal health status. Thus, Dworkin's prudent insurers bear some resemblance to Rawls's original contractors and to the agents of Daniels's "Prudential Lifespan Account," and they share some of the same weaknesses. Dworkin knows these conditions are unrealistic, but he claims they are imaginable, that persons can hypothetically project themselves into this idealized context and ask what standards of care they would choose.

I believe this is a useful intellectual exercise, helpful in encouraging us to break the grip of the rescue principle and the American infatuation with medical miracles. Difficulties arise, however, as we return from these visionary conditions to the present world, which is marked by a widening inequality in income, popular ignorance and overzealousness about the effectiveness of medical interventions, and anxiety about personal health status. Dworkin's ideal prudent purchaser is a useful device for thinking, but in Hume's terms it is still "mere philosophical fiction."[3]

I do not find that thinking from idealized assumptions motivates me to accept change with anything like the force of facing my own vulnerability and recognizing that others are in the same leaky lifeboat with me. This is why I have repeatedly emphasized in this volume the need to wake up to the precariousness of our situation, to place the I in a We context, and to acknowledge a common self-interest in universal care. It is this sort of thinking, I contend, which is the lasting impetus for change. It is this sort of thinking that will finally get us over our romance with rescue and set us free to embrace a more limited, but universal, health care system.

Notes

Index

Notes

Introduction

1. Total health expenditures figures for 1992 are the March 1993 figures from the Health Care Financing Administration (HCFA). Estimates for 1994 and beyond are from HCFA and the Congressional Budge Office. See, also, Thomas Bodenheimer, "Underinsurance in America," *New England Journal of Medicine* 327 (1992), pp. 274–278; "A Call for Action," *The Pepper Commission Report, U.S. Bipartisan Commission on Comprehensive Health Care, Final Report* (Washington, D.C.: U.S. Government Printing Office, 1990); E. Friedman, "The Uninsured: From Dilemma to Crisis," *Journal of the American Medical Association* 265 (1991), pp. 2491–2495; Sally T. Burner, Daniel R. Waldo, and David R. McKusick, "National Health Expenditures Projections through 2030," *Health Care Financing Review* 14 (1992), pp. 1 ff.; and White House Domestic Council, *Health Security: The President's Report to the American People* (New York: Simon and Schuster, 1993). For an excellent exposition of the ethical problems in health insurance practices, see Donald W. Light, "The Practice and Ethics of Risk-Rated Health Insurance," *Journal of the American Medical Association* 267 (1992), pp. 2503–2508.

1. Rationing and the Purpose of a Health Care System

1. Eli Ginzberg, "Health Care Reform—Why So Slow?" *New England Journal of Medicine* 322 (May 17, 1990), pp. 1464–1466.

2. See Larry R. Churchill, *Rationing Health Care in America: Perceptions and Principles of Justice* (Notre Dame, Ind.: University of Notre Dame Press, 1987); see also Victor Fuchs, "The 'Rationing' of Health Care," *New England Journal of Medicine* 311 (December 13, 1984), pp. 1572–1573. Henry Aaron and Wil-

liam Schwartz, without a polemical agenda, specify two senses of rationing in "Rationing Health Care: The Choice before Us," *Science* 247 (January 26, 1990), pp. 418 ff.

3. This point is discussed in greater detail in *Rationing Health Care in America*.

4. For this understanding I am indebted to Professor Glenn Wilson.

5. Arthur Barsky, *Worried Sick: Our Troubled Quest for Wellness* (Boston: Little, Brown, 1988), *passim*.

6. Arnold Relman, "Is Rationing Inevitable?" *New England Journal of Medicine* 322 (June 21, 1990), p. 1810.

7. Arnold Relman, "The Trouble with Rationing," *New England Journal of Medicine* 323 (September 27, 1990), pp. 911–913.

8. The argument takes a variety of forms. Sometimes it includes a comparison between bombers and medication, or between expenditures for popcorn and those for some medical treatment. While we may feel outrage over frivolous uses of money and about waste, more generally, it is sometimes hard to see the point of these comparisons. Arguments for more medicine and less defense can at least be joined, but it makes little sense to urge more medicine and less popcorn. Popcorn is not a government expenditure, nor is it ever likely to compromise anyone's personal or family budget.

9. Lester Thurow, "Learning to Say No," *New England Journal of Medicine* 311 (December 13, 1984), p. 1569.

10. Brian Abel-Smith, "Who Is the Odd Man Out? The Experience of Western Europe in Containing the Costs of Health Care," *Milbank Memorial Fund Quarterly* 63 (1985).

11. See H. Gilbert Welsh and Eric B. Larson, "Dealing with Limited Resources," *New England Journal of Medicine* 319 (July 31, 1988), pp. 171–173. See also Aristotle's discussion of proportionality in matters of justice: "the lesser evil is reckoned a good in comparison with the greater evil"; "Nicomachean Ethics," Book V, Chapter 3, translated by W. D. Ross, in *The Basic Works of Aristotle*, edited by Richard McKeon (New York: Random House, 1941), p. 1007.

12. See, for example, Karen Davis and Diane Rowland, "Uninsured and Underserved: Inequities in Health Care in the United States," *Milbank Memorial Fund Quarterly* 61 (1983), pp. 149–176; and Karen Davis, "Inequality and Access to Health Care," *Milbank Quarterly* 69 (1991), pp. 253–274. For an excellent summary of the access problem from a foreign perspective, see Jennifer Dixon, "U.S. Health Care. I: The Access Problem," *British Medical Journal* 305 (1992), pp. 817–819.

13. Thurow, "Learning to Say No," p. 1572.

14. Norman Daniels, *Am I My Parents' Keeper? An Essay on Justice between the Young and the Old* (New York: Oxford University Press, 1988), p. 18.

15. Ibid., p. 66.

16. Norman Daniels, *Just Health Care* (Cambridge: Cambridge University Press, 1985), pp. 42 ff.

17. Daniels, *Parents' Keeper*, p. 81.

18. Ibid., p. 155.

19. Daniel Callahan, *Setting Limits: Medical Goals in an Aging Society* (New York: Simon and Schuster, 1987), p. 116.

20. Ibid., p. 149.

21. Daniels, *Parents' Keeper*, p. 139.

22. Ibid., p. 147.

23. Daniel Callahan, *What Kind of Life: The Limits of Medical Progress* (New York: Simon and Schuster, 1990).

2. Defining a Purpose: Security and Solidarity

1. See A. Lippman, "Led (Astray) by Genetic Maps: The Cartography of the Human Genome and Health Care," *Social Science and Medicine* 35 (1992), pp. 1469–1476.

2. Charles Dougherty, *American Health Care* (New York: Oxford University Press, 1988).

3. Rashi Fein, *Medical Care, Medical Costs* (Cambridge, Mass.: Harvard University Press, 1986), p. v.

4. Daniel Callahan, *What Kind of Life: The Limits of Medical Progress* (New York: Simon and Schuster, 1990), pp. 31–68.

5. Aristotle, "Nicomachean Ethics," Book V, Chapter 3, translated by W. D. Ross, in *The Basic Works of Aristotle*, edited by Richard McKeon (New York: Random House, 1941).

6. Michael Walzer, *Spheres of Justice* (New York: Basic Books, 1983), p. 89.

7. John Rawls, *A Theory of Justice* (Cambridge, Mass.: Harvard University Press, 1971), pp. 302–303.

8. Norman Daniels, *Just Health Care* (New York: Cambridge University Press, 1985), pp. 41–57.

9. Jeremy Bentham, *An Introduction to the Principles of Morals and Legislation* (New York: Penguin Books, 1987).

10. John Stuart Mill, *Utilitarianism* (Indianapolis: Hackett Publishing Company, 1979).

11. Robert Nozick, *Anarchy, State and Utopia* (New York: Basic Books, 1974), pp. 32–33.

12. Robert Sade, "Medical Care as a Right: A Refutation," *New England Journal of Medicine* 285 (1971), pp. 1288 ff.

13. See, for example, Suzanne W. Letsch, Helen C. Lazenby, Katharine R. Levit, and Cathy A. Cowan, "National Health Expenditures, 1991," *Health Care Financing Review* 14 (Winter 1992), and *Academic Medicine and Health Care Reform: Graduate Medical Education* (Washington, D.C.: AAMC, 1993).

3. Self-Interest and Security

1. See Dan E. Beauchamp, "Discussion," *Bulletin of the New York Academy of Medicine* 68 (1992), pp. 185–192, and *The Health of the Republic* (Philadelphia: Temple University Press, 1988); see also Henry Aaron, *Serious and Unstable Condition: Financing America's Health Care* (Washington, D.C.: The Brookings Institute, 1991).

2. See Janet E. O'Keefe, "Health Care Financing: How Much Reform Is Needed?" *Issues in Science and Technology* 8 (1992), p. 42.

3. As cited in Nancy E. Kass, "Insurance for the Insurers: The Use of Genetic Tests," *Hastings Center Report* 22, no. 6 (1992), p. 8.

4. Thomas H. Murray, "Genetics and the Moral Mission of Health Insurance," *Hastings Center Report* 22, no. 6 (1992), p. 14.

5. David Hume, *A Treatise of Human Nature*, 2d ed., edited by L. A. Selby-Bigge and P. H. Nidditch (Oxford: Clarendon Press, 1978), p. 488.

6. Ibid., p. 490.

7. David Hume, *An Enquiry Concerning the Principles of Morals*, 1777 edition (La Salle, Ill.: Open Court, 1966), p. 21. In the *Enquiry* Hume does not call justice on "artificial" virtue, but in other ways his treatment of it is very similar to his earlier formulation in the *Treatise.*

8. Hume, *Treatise of Human Nature*, p. 492.

9. Thomas Hobbes, *Leviathan*, edited by C. B. MacPherson (New York: Penguin Books Ltd., 1968), p. 186.

10. See, for example, Michael Specter's article, "Neglected for Years, TB Is Back with Strains That Are Deadlier," *New York Times*, October 11, 1992, and the subsequent stories on this problem in the *Times*. See also New York City Health Commissioner Margaret Hamburg's "Poverty, Public Health and Tuberculosis Control in New York City: Lessons from the Past," in *Medical Care and the Health of the Poor*, edited by David E. Rogers and Eli Ginzberg (Boulder: Westview Press, 1993); and *The Journal of Law, Medicine and Ethics*, 21:3–4 (1993), edited by Ronald Bayer, Nancy Neveloff Dubler, and Lawrence O. Gostin, which is entirely devoted to the dual epidemics of tuberculosis and AIDS.

11. John Rawls, *A Theory of Justice* (Cambridge, Mass.: Harvard University Press, 1971).

12. See, for example, Alasdair MacIntyre's *After Virtue* (Notre Dame, Ind.: University of Notre Dame Press, 1981), and Michael J. Sandel's *Liberalism and the Limits of Justice* (Cambridge: Cambridge University Press, 1982).

13. Charles J. Dougherty, *American Health Care* (New York: Oxford University Press, 1988), p. 96.

14. Cited in Bob Rae, "In Canada, Health Care Is Not a Commodity," *Raleigh News and Observer* (April 14, 1992), p. 15A.

15. Hume, *Treatise of Human Nature*, p. 493. See also Adam Ferguson, *An Essay on the History of Civil Society* (1767), republished by Edinburgh Uni-

versity Press, 1966. Skepticism about hypothetical state-of-nature arguments is typical of the philosophers of the Scottish Enlightenment.

16. David Hume, *Essays Moral, Political, and Literary,* edited by Eugene Miller (Indianapolis, Ind.: Liberty Classics, 1985), p. 37.

17. Hume, *Treatise of Human Nature,* p. 620.

18. Hume, *Enquiry Concerning the Principles of Morals,* p. 148. Adam Smith used different imagery but conveyed a similar idea when he call benevolence "the ornament which embellishes," while justice he called "the main pillar that upholds the whole edifice." See Smith's *The Theory of Moral Sentiments* (Oxford: Oxford University Press, 1976), p. 86.

19. For an excellent exposition of this and related points, see Lawrence C. Becker's *Reciprocity* (Chicago: University of Chicago Press, 1986), especially pp. 134 ff.

20. Jane J. Mansbridge, "Preface," *Beyond Self-Interest* (Chicago: University of Chicago Press, 1990), p. xii. The spirit of this volume, edited by Mansbridge, is generally in concert with my thesis and my reading of Hume.

21. Robert B. Reich, *The Work of Nations: Preparing Ourselves for 21st Century Capitalism* (New York: Alfred A. Knopf, 1991), p. 278.

4. Affinity and Solidarity

1. Charles Taylor, *Sources of the Self* (Cambridge, Mass.: Harvard University Press, 1989), p. 196. See also the insightful analysis of atomism by Elizabeth H. Wolgast in *The Grammar of Justice,* chap. 1, "A World of Social Atoms" (Ithaca, N.Y.: Cornell University Press, 1987).

2. Amitai Etzioni, "The Responsive Community (I and We)," *American Sociologist* 18 (Summer 1987), p. 146.

3. Charles Taylor, *Philosophical Papers,* vol. 1, "Introduction" (Cambridge: Cambridge University Press, 1985), pp. 5–8.

4. Rene Descartes, "Meditations," part 4, in *The Philosophical Works of Descartes,* vol. 1, translated by Elizabeth S. Haldane and G. R. T. Ross (Cambridge: Cambridge University Press, 1970), p. 101.

5. David Hume, *A Treatise of Human Nature,* 2d ed., edited by L. A. Selby-Bigge and P. H. Nidditch (Oxford: Clarendon Press, 1978), p. 363.

6. Ibid., pp. 316, 618, 363.

7. Ibid., p. 319.

8. Ibid., p. 365.

9. Ibid., p. 576.

10. Ibid., p. 319; see also p. 386.

11. Ibid., pp. 576, 371.

12. Adam Smith, *The Theory of Moral Sentiments,* edited by D. D. Raphael and A. L. Macfie (Indianapolis: Liberty Classics, 1982), p. 10.

13. Ibid., p. 9.

14. Ibid., p. 21.

15. Ibid., p. 317.

16. Ibid., p. 22.

17. Ibid., p. 112.

18. Maurice Merleau-Ponty, *Phenomenology of Perception*, translated by Colin Smith (London: Routledge & Kegan Paul, 1962), p. 362.

19. James Madison, "Federalist 10," in Alexander Hamilton, James Madison, and John Jay, *The Federalist Papers* (New York: Mentor, 1961), p. 78.

20. David Hume, "Of Parties in General," in *Essays Moral, Political and Literary*, edited by Eugene Miller (Indianapolis: Liberty Classics, 1985), p. 58. See also the insightful analysis of Hume's ideas about factions by Stephen Holmes, "The Secret History of Self-Interest," in *Beyond Self-Interest*, edited by Jane J. Mansbridge (Chicago: University of Chicago Press, 1990), pp. 267–286.

21. Derek L. Phillips, *Looking Backward: A Critical Appraisal of Communitarian Thought* (Princeton, N.J.: Princeton University Press, 1993), p. 167.

5. Rights and Responsibilities

1. President's Commission for the Study of Ethical Problems in Medicine and Biomedical and Behavioral Research, *Securing Access to Health Care: The Ethical Implications of Differences in the Availability of Health Services*, vol. 1 (Washington, D.C.: U.S. Government Printing Office, 1983), p. 4. By contrast, see the excellent exploration of the place of rights in health care reform by Audrey R. Chapman, *Exploring a Human Rights Approach to Health Care Reform* (Washington, D.C.: American Association for the Advancement of Science, 1993).

2. Louis Harris, *Inside America* (New York: Vintage Books, 1987), p. 40.

3. "Making Difficult Health Care Decisions," Louis Harris and Associates for the Harvard Community Health Plan Foundation and the Loran Commission (June 1987), p. 8.

4. Larry R. Churchill, *Rationing Health Care in America: Perceptions and Principles of Justice* (Notre Dame, Ind.: University of Notre Dame Press, 1987), pp. 94 ff.

5. Tom Beauchamp and Ruth Faden, "The Right to Health and the Right to Health Care," *Journal of Medicine and Philosophy* 4 (June 1979), pp. 121–122.

6. Earlier versions of the Good Behavior and the Response models can be found in "Realigning Our Thinking in Health Care: What Are Our Rights and Responsibilities?" *North Carolina Insight* 13 (November 1991), pp. 109–113, and in "Aligning Rights and Responsibilities," a paper prepared for the American Association for the Advancement of Science Right to Health Care Project, December 1992.

7. See *Healthy People 2000: National Health Promotion and Disease Prevention Objectives*, DHHS Pub. No. (PHS) 91–50213 (Washington, D.C.).

8. Dan E. Beauchamp, "Public Health as Social Justice," *Inquiry* 13 (1976), pp. 4–6.

9. An earlier version of the idea of patients and physicians as citizens was developed in relation to patient autonomy and care at the end of life. See Marion Danis and Larry R. Churchill, "Autonomy and the Common Weal," *Hastings Center Report* 21 (January/February 1991), pp. 25–31.

10. See Talcott Parsons, *The Social System* (New York: Free Press of Glencoe, 1951), pp. 428–447.

11. A notable exception to the pattern can be found in Edmund Pellegrino and David Thomasma, *A Philosophical Basis of Medical Practice* (New York: Oxford, 1981), p. 218. Pellegrino and Thomasma list five "patient obligations," yet judicious use of health care resources is not among them.

12. Norman Daniels, *Am I My Parents' Keeper? An Essay on Justice between the Young and the Old* (New York: Oxford University Press, 1988), especially chaps. 3 and 4.

13. Daniel Callahan, *Setting Limits: Medical Goals in an Aging Society* (New York: Simon and Schuster, 1988), especially chap. 5.

14. See "Principles of Medical Ethics," Proceedings of the American Medical Association House of Delegates, 129th Annual Convention, 20–24 July 1980.

15. See the appendix to vol. 4 of *The Encyclopedia of Bioethics*, edited by Warren T. Reich (New York: The Free Press, 1978), pp. 1737–1746.

16. Michael Walzer, *Spheres of Justice* (New York: Basic Books, 1983), p. 89.

17. Norman Daniels, "Why Saying No to Patients in the United States Is So Hard: Cost-Containment, Justice, and Provider Autonomy," *New England Journal of Medicine* 314 (May 22, 1986), pp. 1381–1383.

A Concluding Image

1. Ronald Dworkin, "Will Clinton's Plan Be Fair?" *New York Review of Books*, January 13, 1994.

2. See my discussion of the problems of succumbing to a rescue ethic in *Rationing Health Care in America* (Notre Dame, Ind.: University of Notre Dame Press, 1987), pp. 32–37, 126–128.

3. David Hume, *A Treatise of Human Nature*, 2d ed., edited by L. A. Selby-Bigge and P. H. Nidditch (Oxford: Clarendon Press, 1978), p. 493.

Index